SH*T

THEY DON'T TELL YOU IN NURSING SCHOOL

Jessica Smith Dos Santos, BSN

Cover design by Sean B. with Blissbranding Agency
Published in the United States of America by Jessica Smith Dos Santos, BSN
Hardcover ISBN: 979-8-9894555-3-9
Paperback ISBN: 979-8-9894555-0-8
eBook ISBN: 979-8-9894555-1-5
Audiobook: ISBN: 979-8-9894555-2-2
Library of Congress Control Number: 2023921143
Connect with Jessica at: https://linktr.ee/jessicasmithdossantos

CONTENTS

BEGINNING WITH GRATITUDE

This book would not have been possible without an army of love and support.

Thank you to my loving husband, Jose Luiz, and my incredible teenagers, Gavin and Hailey. You have stood by me, encouraged me, and patiently loved me through the FOUR years it took for this book to come to fruition. You sacrificed time with me so that I may write and you stood steadfast in the belief that this book would serve mankind, even when I had doubts. I love you so much.

Thank you to my dad, Ken, and my mom, Karen, for the childhood of both peace and chaos that shaped me into the woman I am today. Thank you for the love, support, and encouragement that you continue to pour into my life. I would not change a single thing about the life you have given me. I love you and appreciate you.

Thank you to my late Grandma Maylou for speaking inspiration, love, belief, and worth into me at every opportunity. I reflect on all the conversations we have had about our shared desire to write a book and it has given me the courage to continue. I miss you and I wish you were here to celebrate this moment with me. Please pass on a hug to Grandpa and God for me.

Many thanks my dear friend, Jolene Gurney, and her family. Your influence in my life has been immense. You have shown me love, opened my heart and my mind, and walked beside me in this journey of life through many ups and downs. I love you guys!

To Isabel Lerma, my writing coach: This book would not have been possible if it weren't for your writing process. You helped to heal my heart. You found strength, courage, and depth in my writing style that I would not have been able to discover on my own. Thank you for sitting with me in the pain and through the tears, for showing me love and encouragement, and for exposing the story within me so that I could share it with the world.

To Shelley Henk, my coach, mentor, and friend. Partnering with you in health, business, and life has been one of the best decisions I have ever made. You have been steadfast and consistent in your faith in me and your belief in the mission I was put here to serve. You continue to speak hope and encouragement into my life. I am so grateful for you!

To Lizette Balsdon, my editor. If I had known what a process it would be to edit a book I may not have ever started writing. Your guidance, suggestions, and support made the editing process easy and fun. Thank you for your skill and your patience.

Thank you to Megy Davis, esteemed author, mentor, and friend. You have been an answer to prayer and a blessing to my life. You have been so gracious with your time, your care, and your mentorship. Your "pro tip" to listen to my book being read out loud as a part of the editing process saved my bacon! My life is better because you are in it!

Many thanks to Samantha Schwartz-Lenhart and Sean B with Blissbranding Agency for your time and creativity. Your advice and guidance on how to take a book to the market has been invaluable. Extra thanks to Sean, graphics specialist, for the perfect cover design. You were so patient and accommodating with all my ideas and modification requests. I remember you telling me that you were committed to making sure I loved the final product. You fulfilled at a level above and beyond expectation and I appreciate the work you do!

Thank you to the profession of Nursing for teaching me, growing me, breaking me, and inspiring me. Had it not been for the mess you gave me; I would not have a message today. Had it not been for the pain you provided; I would not have the passion and the purpose to serve nurses that I have now. Thank you.

To my fellow Nurses, thank you for your courage and your desire to continue serving our communities across the world. You are the heartbeat of healthcare.

The greatest thanks of all be to God. You planted the seeds of a mission in my heart. You gave me a life path of support that fertilized and watered that mission. You also gave me challenges and trials that taught me, strengthened me, and caused that mission to break free and grow. I know there is so much more yet to come and I am ready for what is next.

SHIT, PISS, AND PUKE: EVERY NURSE'S INITIATION TO THE PROFESSION

Did you know that there are 3 phases of initiation before you are even a "real" nurse? I didn't either.

I was actually initiated into the profession before I had an RN behind my name. I started off my nursing career as a Certified Nurse's Assistant (CNA). Schooling was easy and I figured it was a good way to get my foot in the door of healthcare and to gain experience while I went to nursing school. As with most things in Nursing, I discovered the 3 phases of initiation the hard way: innocent and uneducated experience.

Phase One of Initiation: Shit

I will never forget the elderly man that began my initiation. He was cranky old man with a reputation for being meaner than a junkyard dog. He had not had one single visitor and we were warned that he liked to throw things at the staff. He was sent to the hospital from his group home by ambulance several days prior for chest pain. He was still in the hospital because the group home refused to take him back. Apparently, his behavior was too abusive for their facility. The social worker was trying to find a new place for him to be discharged to; until then, he was ours.

Being a naive optimist, my heart hurt a little hearing his story. What a sad life he must live. I decided then and there that I was going to try to brighten his day and give him a reason to smile. I walked into his room, pushing the vitals machine with one hand, and balancing his breakfast tray in the other. I smiled my best smile and offered a cheery, "Good morning! I brought you some breakfast!"

He looked at me and growled, like an angry caged animal. I continued cautiously toward him; my head cocked to the side as his appearance drew my attention. His teeth were yellow and dirty. His face was leathered and evil. His eyes were filled with contempt; his loathing palpable.

The air felt heavy and thick and the shift in the atmosphere made me stop dead in my tracks. I had never experienced this kind of pure hatred before. Ever. He was scrawny. His arms were bony; his dry and weathered skin hung from his skeleton. His long and thin fingers ended in thick, yellowed, claw-like nails. He actually looked feral and inhospitable. I started to realize that the night shift staff withheld some details in their description of him at the change of shift report.

I immediately felt like an idiot for imagining that I could make his day. As a matter of fact, I understood right away that this man lived a miserable existence. It was as if abominable had become his identity and to crack that persona even a millimeter, would surely mean a swift death.

"Bring me my fucking breakfast," he snarled.

I rocked back on my heels, my eyes wide, feeling as though I had just been slapped. I had heard plenty of language in my life, but no one had ever spoken to me that way, directly. I was simultaneously shocked and insulted. Part of me wanted to tell him off and the other part of me wanted to tuck my tail and run away as fast as I could.

I was dumbfounded, speechless. My feet were frozen to the floor as if trapped in concrete. We stayed silent; eyes locked in a stare-down. It was as if we were in a standoff, both with hands poised above the grips of loaded guns; one waiting for the other to make a move so we could end this scene.

Finally, my chest exhaled the air that was trapped inside, and my feet began to move slowly toward him. Without breaking eye contact, I set the breakfast tray on his bedside table and reached for the blood pressure cuff.

"Don't even think you are going to touch me with that, Sweetie," he snapped.

"Yes, sir," I replied.

My brows furrowed with confusion as I exhaled further. He had verbally slapped me and then called me Sweetie. I was confused. I began slowly backing out of the room.

Something was very wrong with this man. I remembered the comment from the night shift that he liked to throw things at the staff. I was not about to turn my back on him. Out in the hall, I let the nurse know that he had refused to have his vital signs taken. My body felt jittery, as though I had drunk too much coffee. He had invaded my headspace hard and fast, and I was still trying to process what I had just witnessed.

When it was time to collect the empty breakfast trays, I glanced at the door of his room and hesitated. Was this the day a patient was going to throw a fork at me? I took a deep breath and reminded myself that I had been raised on a ranch. I was a sturdy farm girl. I had been kicked by horses, bitten by dogs, attacked by geese and scratched by cats. I was plenty tough and I was not about to let this feral old bag of bones intimidate me. I took a deep breath, squared my shoulders, and went back into the room with some authority in my step.

To my surprise, no fork flew through the air—no, it was much worse!

He sarcastically sneered at me. I detected a small sparkle of glee in his eyes. Again, I was confused by this man. Then it hit me, like a wave crashing its way onto the shore. The putrid smell of sulfur, rotten eggs, skunk, decaying produce, and decomposed meat. My face wrinkled in disgust at the odiferous insult. My shoulders sagged in defeat as my eyes landed on the source of the smell.

In an instant, the meaning of his face became clear. He had removed the plastic plate cover off of his breakfast tray, shit in it, and set it on his bedside table next to his half-eaten breakfast. His sneer was in anticipation of my reaction.

What the hell was wrong with him?

"I had to shit and I wanted to leave you a little present, Sweetie." He delighted in the condescending words.

What an ASS!

My eyes narrowed and I glared at him, my spine stiffening. My happy, optimistic heart turned to stone in an instant. I was done playing nice. Quite frankly, I was pissed. I thought to myself, "Ok, you want to play? Game on, Old Man."

I put on some gloves, calmly walked over to his table, and removed everything except the plastic plate cover with his morning turd sitting in it. I moved the tray table just out of his reach, but still well within sniffing distance. With one last glare and a sarcastic smile of my own, I turned on my heels and started walking out of the room. When he realized that I did not intend to take his prize with me, he began shouting; "Hey! Aren't you going to get that shit out of here!?"

I paused at the door, only half glancing at him over my shoulder, and said, "Nope!"

I walked quickly out the door and out of sight. I would not give him the dignity of an opportunity to respond. I had decided that he could enjoy his disgusting brown steaming present until I was done collecting all the rest of the breakfast trays. I realized that I couldn't leave it there all day and I would eventually have to go back and face the music; but for now, I felt pretty proud of myself.

The war was not over, but I won that battle. Feral bag of bones: Zero. Me: One. I enjoyed a smug little smile as I heard him continue to holler unintelligibly down the hall.

Phase one of initiation: complete.

Phase Two of Initiation: Piss

I went to work feeling fancy and fresh because I had just bought some new work shoes. They were lightweight and felt great on my feet. I hoped that they would be comfortable for the whole 12 hours, unlike my old shoes which were broken down and made my feet hurt about halfway through the shift.

I was walking down the hall, that little extra pep in my step that only comes from that new shoe feel, when I noticed a call light on. It was the sweet little woman I had enjoyed caring for the day before. My mouth turned up at the edges with a little smile as I remembered how kind she was. As I walked in the door, she smiled sweetly at me. She reminded me so much of my grandma. She was a little plump and had full, rosy cheeks. Her smile was kind and her eyes sparkled. Her brownish-gray hair was tinted purple from the hair dye she used. She sported a disheveled, hospital bedhead look that made me grin in a way that felt almost maternal. She was just a joy.

"I'm sorry to bother you, but I have to use the restroom," she said.

I smiled kindly at her and replied, "No problem. I can help you."

I put on some gloves and grabbed the gait belt that was hanging over the foot of the bed. She was still recovering her strength and she remained a little weak in the knees. She had been instructed to call for help to get out of bed as a precaution to protect her from falling. She still needed assistance to stand up and pivot to the bedside commode, because she was not yet able to walk safely to the bathroom. I helped her sit at the side of the bed and positioned the gait belt around her waist.

"Ok, Dear, on the count of three, push up with your legs and pivot over to the commode, just like we did yesterday. One, two, three!"

I shifted my weight back in a staggered squat position to protect my back as she pushed up with her legs, preparing to pivot when all of a sudden, her strength gave out and she lurched forward, her parted legs straddling my thigh. Her hands flailed, desperately grabbing my upper arms as she tried to balance herself. I inhaled sharply and my breath caught in my chest. My muscles contracted, all of my senses hyper-alert. I let out a grunt at the unexpected burden of her full body weight on my thigh. I was instantly flushed. My armpits were damp and a dew of sweat was starting to form in my hairline just above my forehead. The back of my neck radiated with heat.

We were face to face now. Her hands white-knuckle gripping my upper arms, her nails digging into my flesh in terror, afraid to fall. I could smell her morning breath, musty and rancid in my nostrils. I glanced past her shoulder back at the hospital bed, hoping that the emergency call light was close enough for me to activate help.

That's when it happened.

My eyes widened with surprise as she said, "Ooh! Ooh, my God! I can't make it stop!"

My mind scrambled as I tried to make sense of the sensation of warm water flowing down my leg. All at once, everything clicked. My nostrils flared at the realization that my thigh had become her commode.

"I'm so sorry!" Her eyes welled up with tears. Her expression had changed from one of shock to shame. She looked down at the floor, her grip releasing me, her arms sagging against mine in defeat. Embarrassed tears started sliding down her cheeks. Warm urine continued to flow down my leg, my new shoe turning into a squishy, oversaturated sponge. I felt sad for her.

"Hey," I said gently, "Look at me."

She slowly looked up at me, like a child who had been caught doing something wrong. I did my best to smile and lied, "Believe it or not, you are not the first person to pee on me. Just another day on the job over here." I let out a light giggle and she smiled but looked back down at the floor.

"Might as well get it all out so we can get you safely back to bed and cleaned up," I said, trying to sound reassuring. She nodded, still looking down at the floor, as the flow of urine slowed and then came to a stop.

With her cleaned up and tucked safely back into bed, I hesitated at the doorway of her room, looking down at my scrub pants, dark where her urine had flowed down my leg. My mind went to my brand-new shoes.

So much piss.

I wiggled my toes as a way of assessing the situation and I could feel her urine, still warm, sopping between my toes. I took a deep breath and let out a sigh of resignation as I commenced my walk of shame to the nurse's station; each warm, soggy step provoked a soft, squelching sound. So nasty.

Phase two of initiation: complete.

Phase 3 of Initiation: Puke

Why these things always happened at the beginning of a 12-hour shift is beyond me. I think the universe has a cruel sense of humor.

I had just returned to work after a glorious 4 consecutive days off and I felt rested and relaxed. I had woken up a little early that morning and decided to curl my hair and go the extra mile with my makeup. I should have known better. In retrospect, I realize that I was tempting the fates.

I had been making the morning rounds and was headed into the 4-bed ward at the end of the hall for vital signs. As I walked in the door, I made eye contact with the man in the far back corner. Immediately, I knew something was wrong.

He was a middle-aged man, with a large pooch of a belly protruding from under his hospital gown. He was sitting up on the edge of his bed, legs spread wide—leaving nothing to the imagination—bare feet planted on the cold hospital floor. His eyes darted back and forth in front of him, frantically searching. He looked pale and sweaty, and I realized he was about to vomit.

"I'm going to hurl!!!" His words confirmed my suspicions. I rushed toward him, my eyes wildly searching the room for something—anything—I could offer him to puke in. My heart pounded so hard that I could hear it in my ears. I knew there was only a matter of seconds before vomit was coming. My eyes landed on a pink wash basin sitting at the foot of his bed. Without breaking stride, I seized it, recklessly securing the sides of the vessel with both of my hands, arms fully extending to meet him.

He vomited with so much force, it was as if I was witnessing an exorcism. Rancid chunks of puke hit the bottom of the basin and ricocheted right back out. I barely had time to close my eyes and my mouth as a pressure hose of hot, putrid vomit hit my pretty face, my cute curled hair, my fresh scrub top. It was all I could do to keep from gagging in my own mouth. I was engulfed. When the onslaught was over, I slowly wiped the warm, fetid slime off my face with my bare hand and opened my eyes. There was a little fleck of leftover stomach content hanging from my eyelash, which I wiped away with my other bare hand.

What the actual fuck just happened?

I stood there, staring at him in total and utter shock, my jaw clenched, afraid to inhale. He looked back at me, jaw hanging open, dribbles of vomit dripping off his stubbled chin and down the front of his gown.

Oh. My. God.

I set the puke-filled basin on his lap without saying a word and walked over to the sink. I began furiously washing myself with hot water and copious amounts of soap from the soap dispenser. When I finally dared to look at myself in the mirror, my face bright red, taut, and strained from scrubbing with hospital hand soap, I took note that my mascara had run down my cheeks and I looked like a drowned raccoon. I smelled even worse. My beautiful curls were matted together with vomit and clinging to the side of my neck like slimy leeches.

With the adrenaline from the assault wearing off, I just wanted to cry. No more cute curls. Extra mile makeover ruined. I should have just let him puke all over the floor. This was revolting and humiliating. I felt like a dirty sewer rat and couldn't get the smell of puke out of my nostrils. It was going to be a long day.

Phase three of initiation: complete.

Why I still thought I wanted to be a nurse after that is beyond me. I guess I figured that since I had already been initiated, I might as well get properly compensated. Truth is, initiation gave me the foresight to have a clean set of scrubs, undergarments, shoes, and shower supplies in my locker at all times.

Why the hell didn't they tell us that in nursing school?

Real Talk

5-minute writing prompt:
Write about your shit, piss, or puke story. Pick one or do all three!

Reality Check

As nurses, we expect to have encounters with shit, piss, and puke. What we don't always expect is HOW these encounters will happen. What's more challenging is that we are never prepared for how we may react to it! We are unsuspectingly triggered and left to wonder WTF just happened. It is moments like this that I wish I knew then what I know now.

Take Action

Join the S**t They Don't Tell You in Nursing School community and share your shit, piss, and puke stories with us! We would love to hear all the unexpected ways you got dumped on!

Scan QR code to join

https://linktr.ee/jessicasmithdossantos

BEFORE WE CONTINUE

Before we continue, there are a few things I think you should know. This book is for the new nurse just starting out in the dynamic career of Nursing. It is also for the Nurse who may be facing disappointment, discouragement, or burnout, and is looking to revive his or her passion for the vocation. More than anything, this book is for the Nurse who recognizes that if nothing changes, nothing changes.

In a medical model that was only ever designed to react to disease, this book serves to disrupt the way you, my fellow Nurse, experience the stress of the career. The purpose of this book is to empower, prepare, and support Nurses to first and foremost be their own greatest caregivers so that they may feel alive, fulfilled, and fully aligned.

I share vulnerably from the heart: my personal guilt, my shame, my fear, my anger, my self-judgment, my addictions to food, and my struggles with alcohol are on the table for all to witness. I have been given a path to healing that has taken years of education, support, therapy, community, and dedication to coaching to become the balanced, aligned, inspired woman I am today. Now, it is my responsibility to pay it forward to you.

If you are hurting in the ways that I was, I hope my stories let you know that you are not alone. If you are feeling emotionally vulnerable and raw right now, I want you to know that there is hope. There is a better way.

If at any point you are triggered as you read this book, please stop and skip directly to the PAUSE THE HUSTLE section of the book. PAUSE THE HUSTLE is a tool that provides simple steps to assist with processing the emotions that may be present for you.

While the stories contained in this book are based on my personal experiences, the names and identifying facts of events have been altered with fictional details and characters in accordance with HIPPA laws to protect personal information as well as to maintain the integrity of the medical systems and to honor the talented staff that serves in them. The only exception to this rule is Lauren's story. I have the blessing of her family to share her real name and her story as a part of this book.

If you are a non-medical professional, consider yourself warned. While this book will provide plenty of entertainment value, lessons, and tools that will be helpful to you too, it also contains vivid descriptions of the human condition, illnesses, bodily fluids, and behavior that may be disturbing to you.

Like the cover of this book says: It is real, it is raw, and I hold nothing back.

I am willing to let it all hang out so that the brokenness that exists in the profession can be exposed for what it is, and we can join together as a community to become the solution we all desperately need.

I always tell my clients: Life doesn't get less hard; we just learn how to do hard better. With a little work and the right support in place, you can empower yourself to become your own liberator.

Please don't stop at just reading this book; decide right now to take what you learn and implement it in your daily life.

Much Love,

Coach Jess

WHY DID YOU BECOME A NURSE?

Why did you become a Nurse?

I became a nurse because I love people.

This is, and always has been, the core of what I was put here on this Earth to do: love people.

When I decided to become a nurse, I was a 17-year-old senior in high school with a pocket full of dreams, and my future in the palms of my hands. I knew I loved to help people. I also knew that nurses helped people. I indulged in daydreaming about wearing scrubs, saving lives, and making a difference in the world.

I imagined what it would be like to make a living only working 3 days a week. My chest swelled with pride as I pictured in my mind's eye all of the people who would be so proud of me for getting my nursing degree. My parents, my grandparents, my professors… I envisioned being head-over-heels in love with my profession. I dreamed about all of the people who would be so grateful for me; so thankful for the care I gave them, so happy to have met me.

Twinkles in my eyes, smiles on my cheeks, pockets full of sunshine.

Nursing school was a brutal 2 years. I worked full-time as a CNA all the way through nursing school. I spent many late nights filling out medication cards, typing up care plans, and scouring over nursing diagnoses. There were long clinical rotations, and I studied until I couldn't keep my eyes open.

In spite of the grind, I remained optimistic and full of anticipation. I imagined the inspiring things I would get to do, as the badass nurse I would become, and the life I would afford myself because of this incredible career choice.

I started off my speech as Salutatorian of the nursing class of 2005 with, "I didn't choose nursing, nursing chose me," and I meant every word.

Where It All Began

Let me take you back to when I was seven. I stood in the living room, my skinned knees peeking out of the holes in my jeans. I rocked my favorite Rainbow Brite tank top, my tangled hair pulled back in a messy self-made side ponytail.

My 7-year-old heart was so worried about my Dad. He had recently had his vasectomy and he was still walking funny. His knees were bowed out to the sides and his steps were much shorter and more careful than usual. He was hunched over a little bit. He looked as though he was in pain.

He had traded his usual blue jeans for a baggy pair of sweatpants for the third day in a row. Dad never wore sweatpants in the middle of the day. Concern furrowed my eyebrows and painted a skeptical frown on my lips.

I knew I was going to be a nurse someday, and I also knew plenty about infections. I had been born and raised on a ranch and I had seen enough animals with infected wounds in my 7 years of life. I was practically an expert, and I was quite certain that my dad had an infection from his surgery.

"Hey, Dad," I asked.

"Yeah," he replied.

"You look pretty bad," I said.

"I'm ok." He tried to give me a reassuring smile, but I wasn't having it.

"I don't think so. I think you have an infection."

"No, I don't. I'm just still a little sore from the surgery."

"Do you have an incision?"

"Yes. But a very very small one."

"I think it is infected," I asserted, certain that he had an infection.

"I promise. I don't have an infection."

"Can I inspect your incision to make sure?" I knew you had to keep a close eye on these things and I just didn't trust that he knew what he was talking about.

"I don't think so."

"Why not?" I kept pressing, my tone rising slightly.

"Well, because it is a very sensitive, private area. It is not a spot that is appropriate to share with other people."

"But you shared it with the Doctor. Besides, I am going to be a nurse someday and I should probably check it out."

"Not today, kiddo."

I sighed, glaring at him. "Did you have to get stitches?"

"Yes, but only 1 or 2."

"Hmm. Are you sure you don't have an infection? I can check." My eyes widened with hope and I was nodding my head up and down.

"You don't need to check. I have to go back to the Doctor tomorrow and they will check it there to be sure. Thanks though." He held his arms out inviting me in for a hug.

I was doubtful; but I leaned in and tightly wrapped my arms around him. I might not have been able to inspect the incision, but I wasn't going to take my eyes off of him.

The next 24 hours felt like YEARS to my worried 7-year-old mind. I sat on the front porch anxiously waiting for him to come home from his follow-up appointment the next day. My bare feet bounced up and down on the wooden planks, my little fingers fidgeted in my lap. When I saw the car pulling into the driveway, I shot off the porch and sprinted down the dirt driveway, naked feet kicking up dust and rocks as my little legs ran. I could see his face smiling at me through the windshield as the car met me about halfway. The car had barely slowed to a stop as I yanked open the passenger side door and jumped into the seat.

"Well?" I questioned between gasps of air.

He didn't say a word but instead, handed me a piece of folded-up gauze. I opened it carefully and was delighted to see two little black sutures sitting in the middle. My face radiated with relief. The sutures were out! I looked back at him and smiled.

"No infection," he smiled.

I scooched across the bench seat and wrapped my arms around him.

Even then, I was fascinated by the human condition. I was naturally drawn to and in tune with injury and suffering. I loved the feeling of assisting in the process of recovery. There has always been an essence in me that is like the secret ingredient of a family recipe. An essence that can't be qualified or quantified, but which we all have in common. The essence of a Nurse.

I didn't choose nursing, nursing chose me. I believed, deep in my being, that I was made for this purpose. Nursing was my calling.

I had seen the older nurses during my clinical rotations, smiling and shaking their heads with that all-knowing "look" when I shared my eager enthusiasm with them. Despite my air of innocence and their apparent skepticism, I was determined to make a difference.

The day I received the news that I had passed the NCLEX, I was so freaking proud of myself. I had done it! All that grueling work in nursing school had finally paid off.

I was now Jessica Smith, BSN, RN. With those letters behind my name, I felt free.

Little did I know, that feeling of freedom was nothing but a well-curated fantasy. The long, weary nights of preparing for clinicals were nothing compared to the exhaustion I would later feel. I had no idea that the emotional overwhelm of fear, disgust, shame, guilt, resentment, heartbreak, disappointment, and doubt, would eventually wear me down and lead to hard-core burnout.

I would not have been able to fathom the idea that my optimistic heart—full of hope and determination—would grow hard and weary. I didn't think that the difficult days would find me naked in the shower, drinking wine, and eating chocolate; crying until there were no more tears to cry.

I would never have predicted that I would beg to stop feeling and I would turn to bourbon—straight out of the bottle—to numb out the emotions. I never knew that when I thought I had nothing left to give, I would be required to give even more.

Holidays, school events, vacations, family dinners, birthdays, anniversaries—NOTHING was sacred and everything was contingent on employer approval.

I often caught myself wondering, "Why did I decide to become a nurse?"

As I reflect back on this question, I realize that I became a nurse based on a fantasy of what I thought nursing would be like. I was a naive, optimistic, 17-year-old with my whole life ahead of me. A virgin of the world, full of hope and in pursuit of my best life. My 17-year nursing career turned into an education on the realities of how things really worked in nursing.

No doubt, this profession is dynamic. It is filled with joy and heartache, wins and losses, highs and lows, extreme happiness and deep sadness, excitement and agony.

Experience taught me that the greater the fantasy in your mind about what you think nursing will be like, the more profoundly shattering the experience of the realities will be for you.

Real Talk

5-minute writing prompt:
Why did you become a nurse?

Reality Check

We each have our own motivations for becoming a Nurse. We might have followed different paths that led us to the same profession, but our hearts, our inspirations, and our motivations allow us to unite in our desire to serve our community. We become family.

Unfortunately, we have also become bonded in our traumas, our burnout, and our dysfunction as a way of coping. Along my journey to healing, I learned that having the RIGHT community surrounding me was incredibly important. I had to be willing to stop commiserating with my peers about all that was wrong and start being willing to have conversations about how I could take personal responsibility for my experiences. As a first step to connecting to a healthy community, I invite you to follow me on Facebook for inspiration, stories of reclaiming health and happiness, nutritious recipes, tips on increasing happiness, improving physical health, having better relationships, and more.

Take Action

We would love to get to know you more! If you haven't already, join the Sh*t They Don't Tell You in Nursing School community.

We are a community of Nurses who are ready do Nursing differently, and we are looking forward to hearing your thoughts!

Scan QR code to join

https://linktr.ee/jessicasmithdossantos

MY STORY

You might be wondering, who is this chick? How is she even qualified to be writing this book?

Well, I am a retired Registered Nurse (RN) with a Bachelor's Degree in Science, emphasis in Nursing (BSN). My first few years in telemetry led me to an Advanced Cardiac Life Support Certification (ACLS). Later in my 17-year career, I transitioned into a level 2 trauma center emergency room. I worked my way through cross-training in all the roles in the emergency department; starting with the lower acuity patients and triage and working my way up to the highest acuity patients, trauma, and even the trauma team lead and charge nurse roles.

Working in trauma required additional certification through the Trauma Nursing Core Course (TNCC). I primarily worked with adults, but I also occasionally floated over to the pediatric ER. I enjoyed pediatrics and I loved teaching, so I obtained certification as an Emergency Nurse Pediatric Course (ENPC) instructor. I took my career seriously and went on to acquire national Board Certification as an Emergency Nurse (BCEN).

Seventeen years of service to my community, five years of formal education, and thousands of dollars invested in degrees and certifications earned me the title: Jessica Smith, BSN, RN, BCEN, ENPC-I. If we are looking at credentials as qualifications to write this book, I would say I am severely overqualified.

But now, I have evolved to become Jessica Smith Dos Santos, full-time owner, CEO, and Transformation Coach of my own coaching practice, which costed thousands of additional dollars and many more years invested in learning the crafts of coaching and business. I have been personally coached and mentored in health and in business since 2014. I have coached over one thousand clients in their own transformation. I leverage a physician-led system for physical, mental, and financial health that is unparalleled in simplicity and results. I personally mentor coaches to both launch and scale their coaching practices and I have co-curated a team of coaches who serve a dedicated group of clients as a collective to create lives that they love to live. I retired my nursing license and the rush of saving lives in the ER to invest in the joy of business ownership and human transformational technology. Instead of saving lives, I empower people to save their own lives.

But all of those are just titles, information, and letters behind a name. Truth be told, not one of those things uniquely qualifies me to be sharing my story or offering you any comfort, hope, wisdom, advice, or strategies.

So why bother continuing to read this book?

Because I am you. I have been in the trenches of nursing. I have done and seen things that were never covered in nursing school. I have experienced burnout, moral injury, and compassion fatigue. I was never given any tools to support myself in finding my way through. I developed a bad attitude. I started feeling like the victim of a profession that lied to me about what nursing was really like in the real world. I was resentful at the time and money I had invested to have all those letters behind my name. I remember feeling betrayed when I finally realized that I had been sheltered from the realities of this career. I eventually understood that being fully engaged in the profession also meant sacrificing important things like relationships, physical and mental health, sleep, and time with my friends and family. Exhaustion became a normal state of being.

Slowly, over time, I became desensitized and what was once fucking hard, became just another ordinary day. I lost that sense of fulfillment for the work I did and my heart slowly died from the inside out as patient volumes doubled and management became more demanding.

One day, I woke up burned-out, depleted, and bitter. I became anxious and tearful at the idea of having to go back to work. I caught myself saying things like, "I hate people," "My soul is dying," and "I can't do this anymore."

I felt lied to and ripped off because I thought I was investing in a career that would bring flexibility, satisfaction, and abundant income. I felt like I had paid to become a prisoner; at the mercy of the hospital's demands for staffing, worked like a dog, and barely paid enough to keep up with inflation.

I felt lied to and ripped off because I thought I had invested in a career that would bring flexibility, satisfaction, and abundant income. I felt like I had paid to become a prisoner; at the mercy of the hospital's demands for staffing, worked like a dog, and barely paid enough to keep up with inflation.

I have the unique perspective of being from a generation of nurses who charted on paper and still had the benefit of enough time in the day to create a relationship with the patients we served. I have experienced the shift from "the good ole days" in nursing to computer charting, checklist protocols, and satisfaction-based reimbursement. I have struggled with the modification of a patient-focused care model to one where productivity and throughput lead the way.

I have been dragged into the depths of burnout, exhaustion, and overwhelm when I had nothing but my own stubborn desire to want better for myself than the reality I was living. Quite frankly, I wasted way too much time believing that the profession of Nursing was the villain of my story.

I dedicated the last 6 years of my nursing career to taking accountability for my experience, seeking a better way, and allowing myself to be humbled by the cold, hard truth that it was my own mindset that created my suffering and kept me trapped. I have devoted years of my life to the craft of coaching and serving others to find their way through.

More than anything, what qualifies me to speak into your journey is the fact that I lost myself completely to the profession of Nursing. I wandered in the void between what I thought I would be doing as a nurse, and the stark reality of what I actually did every day; and, after years of coaching programs and instruction, I found my way back. Bounced back from burnout.

I gave it all up and let it all go for another shot at creating a life designed around what matters most to me.

Out of the pain of the profession, the scars of the losses, and the ashes of burnout, this book was birthed. It is filled with hard truths, difficult stories, and a whole lot of badass love.

That unconditional kind of love that is willing to ask the hard questions and hold space for the hurt, the tears, the frustration, and honesty so that healing may occur. I hope to provide you with tangible experience, lessons from 17 years in the profession, and my best tools to support you in navigating the shit they don't tell you in nursing school. Because the most important thing they didn't tell you in nursing school is that YOU MATTER. Your health, your voice, your well-being, your relationships, your quality of life…YOU. YOU MATTER.

Real Talk

5-minute writing prompt:
What is your story?

Reality Check

We all have stories full of success and failure, joy and heartbreak, happiness and depression and I believe that getting stuck in guilt and shame prevent us from owning our stories in a way that allows our pain to become our purpose and our mess to become our message. Each and every one of us was given a custom curriculum that has brought us to this exact moment in our lives and your story matters.

Take Action

If you are struggling to own your story and are feeling disconnected from your purpose, I offer a complimentary coaching call. It would be my pleasure to support you in seeing your story from a different perspective. Simply scan the QR code, click the "book a free call" link, and schedule a time to connect.

Scan QR code to schedule

https://linktr.ee/jessicasmithdossantos

SHIT THEY DON'T TELL YOU IN NURSING SCHOOL

It's not the blood, the vomit, the feces, the urine, or the sputum that will get to you. Those are the things you expect when you sign up to become a nurse. It will be the shit they don't tell you in nursing school that will shock you, shatter your innocence, rattle your emotions, and make you question why you signed up to be a nurse in the first place.

Shit like:

- How you, yourself, will FEEL your patient's pain, suffering, sadness, devastation, anger, fear, and frustration.
- The shock you will experience when a patient tells you to fuck off as they throw their discharge papers in your face and push you on their way out the door.
- The guilt trips you will get from management begging you to come in for "just one more shift" because they are short-staffed.
- The surprise you will feel when you hear yourself say, "I don't get paid enough for the crap I have to deal with."

- The heartache you will feel as you witness a patient signing DNR paperwork while the family sobs at the bedside.
- The terror you feel when the newly born infant is limp, blue, and lifeless.
- The horror you feel when you realize you have made a mistake that may forever alter a patient's life.
- The feeling of fighting back the tears and trying to breathe around the lump in your throat as you witness the gut-wrenching sobs of the parents whose infant you could not revive after they left her alone near water.
- The overwhelming shitstorm of emotions you go through when caring for an abused child whose injuries are so severe that you are certain the next breath will be the last.
- The anger you harbor at the injustice of what people are capable of doing to one another.
- The mental and emotional fatigue of second-guessing your every move when your patient dies and you know you did not have enough time to try everything you had available.
- The adrenaline that courses through your body when caring for a patient suffering a heart attack, stroke, or trauma. Time is of the essence and everything you do or do not do could mean life or death.
- The anger that permeates your being when you are hit, kicked, punched, slapped, spit at, intentionally urinated on, scratched, bitten, cursed at, and have to dodge things that are being thrown at you. Anger is compounded by the fact that there are minimal consequences for the abuser.
- The resentment that dwells inside of you each time you are denied a request to take time off.

- The nightmares that wake you up in a panicked sweat as you re-live work in your sleep.
- The physical, mental, and emotional exhaustion—the byproducts of long shifts with no breaks, mandatory overtime, and constant multitasking.
- The shock, helplessness, and panic that chills your bones when a Hepatitis C patient's blood splashes in your eye or when you suffer your first contaminated needlestick injury.
- The desperation that breaks your heart when the flashbacks of what you have seen, smelled, touched, and experienced won't stop.
- The gut-wrenching anguish of being so emotionally overwhelmed you can't even stand to be touched by your loved ones or your children. They miss you and want to be with you, but you have nothing left to give, and are too vandalized to receive.
- The numbness that deadens your soul when you are too wrecked to process, and shutting down is all you have left.
- The despair you feel when you realize that this profession is not what you thought you signed up for, and you finally admit that you are burned-out, jaded, and angry. Innocence destroyed.

————————————————————————

Nursing school does not prepare you for the emotional toll this career can have, nor does it equip you with usable strategies to care for yourself when you feel emotionally burned-out. These things come as a shock in the real world, and you quickly comprehend that you do not have the training or the coping skills needed to process the extreme polarity of emotions you will experience.

Nursing school does not prepare you for the emotional toll this career can have, nor does it equip you with usable strategies to care for yourself when you feel emotionally burned-out. These things come as a shock in the real world and you quickly comprehend that you do not have the training or the coping skills needed to process the extreme polarity of emotions you will experience. There is a cost of caring. A price to be paid for what you will do.

As a nurse, you are at high risk for Secondary PTSD, compassion fatigue, moral injury, and burnout. Your patients and their families will look to you for strength and comfort when their worlds fall apart. They don't realize that there is an emotional and physical price that you pay in order to be that strength for them. They don't realize that you will feel the emotional pain right along with them. They don't realize that you may not be equipped to hold that emotional space for them in a way that does not harm your soul, but you will do it anyway. They would never know the price you pay to be their strength, because you become a master at disguising your emotions.

As nurses, we have a front-row seat to human pain and suffering. Sometimes, we have the power—and privilege—to ease that ache. Sometimes, we are powerless and endure emotional agony in the name of our career. Regardless, we have to stay on our toes every moment and continue moving on to the next person who needs our help, and the next, and the next. The need for what we provide never ends. While what we have to give is a resource that takes time to renew, those who need a drink never stop coming.

We develop super-human emotional composure and emotional endurance as strategies to keep up with the demands of the profession, but the mechanisms in which these skills are obtained are soul killers; stuffing the emotions down, binge eating, retail therapy, alcohol, promiscuity, drugs, dark humor. In short, numbing.

Not processing, not coping, not releasing. Numbing.

Cynda Rushton, a professor of clinical ethics and nursing and pediatrics at John Hopkins University, has identified that this type of experience, when continually repeated, can cause nurses to become "angry or hypervigilant or to shut down or numb out so they aren't able to engage." These symptoms in caregivers are now being called Secondary PTSD. I have been in the nursing profession since 2003, and I can relate to being emotionally shut down and unable to engage both at work and in my personal life. I have subscribed to emotional eating, binge drinking, over-exercising, promiscuity, and retail therapy in my attempts to just feel better.

I have faked a cold and called in sick 3 shifts in a row because I could not fathom going back to work. I have caught myself crying on my way to work because I just didn't know if I had it in me to work one more shift. I was never warned that I could be physically abused by my patients just for trying to help. They never told me that patients and their family members are verbally and emotionally abusive.

Unprepared, thrown in the deep end, encouraged to eat candy and pizza when shit was extra hard. Begged to come back for more because short staffing never stops, no matter how many times they promise you it will get better. The fact is, we are taught to hide our emotional pain and "be strong". The price is high; so high that sometimes, the pain of the caring profession we all signed up for is so horrible that suicide seems like the only way out.

I have personally grieved the loss of 4 co-workers who successfully committed suicide in my 17 years of nursing. The loss of someone you have served with, mentored, grown a friendship with, and cared for, leaves a scar on your heart deeper than all the rest

Lauren

Trigger warning: this content may cause some intense emotions. If you are concerned about being triggered, refer to the PAUSE THE HUSTLE section now and at any time throughout this book.

I have personally grieved the loss of 4 co-workers who successfully committed suicide in my 17 years of nursing. The loss of someone you have served with, mentored, grown a friendship with, and cared for leaves a heart scar a little deeper than all the rest.

Let me tell you about Lauren.

When I met her, she had just graduated from nursing school and had fought her way into being hired in the level 2 trauma center emergency room. I was tasked with being her mentor. It was my job to prepare her to be a confident, competent, and independent ER nurse and I had 16 weeks to do it.

For a brand-new graduate nurse, starting in any department in the hospital is daunting; but starting in ER is like jumping into the deep end of the ocean with beginner swimming skills and only a vague idea of what getting caught in a rip tide might feel like. I admired her tenacity and her desire to show up and contend for her dream of being an ER nurse.

Working with Lauren was not an easy task. First of all, our personalities were polar opposites. I am pretty open and bubbly. I love to chat with people and find reasons to laugh. I'm a hugger. I have a mission to collect at least 15 hugs every day. And I smile… a lot.

Lauren, reporting for ER nurse duty, was none of those things. She was rigid, stoic, and serious. She wore this expression on her face that said she was here for business and business only. She always showed up early to her shift with her long, wavy brown hair tied back in a ponytail. The first time I tried to give her a hug, she went stiff as a board, and took a step back to get away from me.

Not a hugger; noted. I remember thinking, "Shit. This is going to be a looong 16 weeks of orientation."

Over the course of our time together, I came to understand that Lauren was fiercely intelligent, had a huge heart that cared for people, did actually love to hug (but only her dog), and she wanted to be the best nurse she could possibly be. Hence the "all business" attitude for 12 hours a day, every day. Lauren felt a huge responsibility to prove herself and grow her skills, because it was rare for a new graduate nurse to be hired in the ER straight out of school.

While I didn't get any hugs and smiles were rare, I came to adore Lauren. She was like the yin to my yang. We developed a flow together; a mentor/new grad dance that started with me leading and her following. We progressively transitioned to her taking the lead and me being the follower. There was such a sense of accomplishment for both of us when she would confidently care for a patient that was once outside of her comfort zone and skill set.

When Lauren grew in her skills and relaxed into her role a bit more, she started opening up. A little. I learned that she loved her dog, Wesley, and that she gave him lots of hugs. I laughed out loud when she told me that he usually stiffened up and tried to get away from her when she went in for a hug—the exact same way she did when I tried to hug her.

I understood that she was a voracious student and thirsted for new knowledge during her time away from the hospital. I discovered that she had huge goals, both personally and professionally. I uncovered the fact that she was a MASSIVE Star Wars fan. She was completely appalled when I confessed that I had never seen any of the Star Wars movies (still haven't), and that I loved the Little Mermaid.

During our 16 weeks of training, we bonded. We saved lives together. We lost lives together. We experienced extreme sadness, intense joy, frustration, anger, happiness, and all the other emotions in between. We had the same victories and the same defeats. We had the same doubts and fears and unanswered questions that come with critically ill patients. We also shared the same sense of friendship.

On our last shift together, she greeted me at the charge desk with a smile and a little gift in her hand. Seeing her smile first thing in the morning was such a rare treasure! She had brought me a coffee mug with Princess Ariel on it that said, "Life is short, make a splash". I felt KNOWN by her, appreciated by her, cared for by her. Of course, I had brought a little gift for her as well. I found a Darth Vader bobble head, and for the first time in 16 weeks, I actually saw her eyes sparkle with joy. I'm pretty sure she felt known, appreciated, and cared for, too. At the end of our shift, I could barely contain myself.

I wanted to give her a hug so badly and she could tell. She smiled and said, "Ok, just this once, you can hug me." It was one of the best hugs of my whole life. I felt honored to have earned that hug and she willingly hugged me back. That hug was the greatest gift she could have ever given me.

I worked day shift and she worked nights, so we rarely saw each other after that. We did keep in touch periodically via text. I would check in on her now and again and the word on the street was that she was doing pretty well. Still taking her job very seriously and desiring to grow in her career.

About a year later (or maybe it was 2? The timeline is a little fuzzy for me at this point), Lauren reached out to me and asked to meet for coffee. I was thrilled to catch up with her in person, as she had changed jobs and went to another hospital. She sat in the chair across from me at the coffee shop, shoulders relaxed, a peaceful expression on her face. She was open, talkative, and seemed to be genuinely settling into her career path and enjoying her profession. She shared stories of her experiences with patients, times that were hard, and times that she was really proud of the work she had done. We chatted for about 30 minutes and when it was time to leave, I received a second hug from her. She leaned in, arms open, inviting me. My heart felt so happy to experience her more relaxed and open.

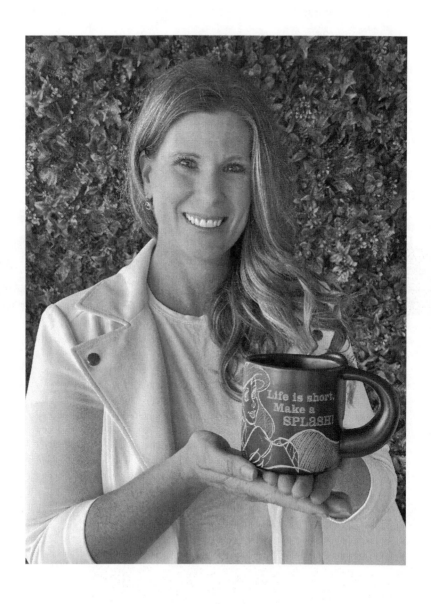

Little did I know, that was the last
hug I would ever receive from Lauren.
About a week later, I learned that she
had successfully committed suicide.

Little did I know, that was the last hug I would ever receive from Lauren. About a week later, I learned that she had successfully committed suicide.

The day I received the news I felt as though I had been gut-punched; doubled-over, trying to catch my breath, as my mind struggled to believe the news was real. When I met her for coffee the week before, she seemed so peaceful and confident. She hugged me, willingly. My chest tightened and my face contorted with tears.

Suicide?

With a lump in my throat and a stream of hot, salty tears rolling down my face, a floodgate of questions bombarded my mind.

Had I missed something?

Was she trying to give me a clue that I didn't catch?

Was she so peaceful because she had already made the decision to end her life and was saying her goodbyes?

Could I have done something differently to support her?

Should I have reached out more often?

Was that hug so genuine because she already knew it would be our last?

Why didn't she tell me she was suffering?

Why didn't she just tell someone?

Was it because our mental health system sucks so bad that she was afraid to seek help?

Oh, my God—her dog. Her parents. My legs turned to noodles and I collapsed on the ground. My shoulders slumped in defeat; my heart cut deep with the sharp knife of a short life as tears continued to stream down my face.

They never told me I might lose a co-worker to suicide. They never told me how bad it would hurt. They never fucking prepared me for this in nursing school.

Losing Lauren left a scar on my heart that was wider and deeper than all the rest. I sometimes sip morning coffee out of the mug she gave me and I reflect on our 16 weeks together. I get tears in my eyes thinking about our last hug. Sometimes, it still feels a little unfair. We were all robbed of a beautiful human with so much potential. If only we had known how deeply she was hurting.

I wish I could tell you that Lauren was the only one that we lost to suicide in the 17 years I served as a nurse, but sadly, she was not.

As a department, we united to support those that had attempted to commit suicide and were on the road to recovery. We also grieved together as a community each time a co-worker's life was lost to suicide. Each loss and near loss rocked us to our core, like an earthquake, reminding us that we are sturdy and yet, we are oh-so fragile.

In my research about nursing and suicide, multiple resources pointed to the fact that nurses were at higher risk for suicidal thoughts than non-nurses. In an article titled "Deaths by Suicide Among Registered Nurses: A Rapid Response Call", authors Katherine A Lee, BSN, RN and Christopher R Friese, PhD, RN, AOCN FAAN (2021) share,

> "Using the latest available data from the Centers for Disease Control and Prevention National Violent Death Reporting System, Davis and colleagues (2021) found that between 2007 and 2018, nurses were 18 percent more likely to die from suicide than the general population. Among female nurses, the risk of death by suicide was nearly twice the risk observed in the general population, and 70 percent

more likely than female physicians ([Davis et al. (2021)](#)) also reported that from 2017 to 2018, an estimated 729 American nurses committed suicide, the highest reported number on record. But we fear the worst is yet to come. The repetitive and traumatic stress experienced during the COVID-19 pandemic has placed nurses at substantially higher risks for poorer mental health, relative to other health professions ([Kunz et al., 2021](#))"

This is not to say that nursing as a profession is to be solely blamed for nurses taking their own lives; but what is certain, is that the job stress of nursing creates a compounded risk of death by suicide. One source called the profession of nursing a "fertile soil for risk of suicide." [ANA]. The theme of a majority of articles addressing the topic of nursing and suicide was the stigma of asking for help and pointed to providing training to identify the signs of suicidal thoughts in our colleagues as a solution. One source even went as far as to say, "We can learn ways to reach nurses in the dark place of depression to reduce the risk of a nurse acting on their suicidal thoughts." [ANA]

But isn't that already too late? We already know that nurses are masters of disguise, so why are we waiting to identify the signs rather than starting at the very beginning? Why not empower nurses with masterful emotional skills while they are in nursing school?

As I reflect on my friend, Lauren, and the other friends lost along the way, I do wonder if their stories would have been different if they were given more skills to navigate their emotions. I wonder if they would have been more resilient had they been given the opportunity to practice emotional processing skills as a part of their clinical experience.

I wonder if they entered the profession with their eyes wide open and knew about the pitfalls of numbing emotions, would they have written a different story? I wonder, how can we do more to empower those who give so much to care for others?

The tools I provide in this book are a single step toward empowering you to take better care of yourself. They are part of the ongoing effort to equip nurses with the knowledge and tools needed to enhance their practice. However, the broader mission of addressing mental health issues among nurses has only just begun. Setting nurses free to be alive, fulfilled and fully aligned so they can feel good about serving others again is of paramount importance to the communities they serve.

Special thanks to Lauren's mom, Dena, for giving me permission to share her story and her real name as part of this book. I continue to send my love and prayers to you and your wonderful family. In honor of her memory, we invite you to donate to the Lauren Delameter Memorial Scholarship fund: https://nvnurses-foundation.org/Donations/[1]

---

[1] **Sources:**
Lee KA, Friese CR (2021). *Deaths by Suicide among Registered Nurses: A Rapid Response Call.* [PubMed]
Davidson JE, Accardi R, Sanchez C, Zisook S, & Hoffman LA (2020). *Sustainability and Outcomes of a Suicide Prevention Program for Nurses. Worldviews on Evidence-Based Nursing, 17(1), 24–31. 10.1111/wvn.12418* [PubMed] [CrossRef] [Google Scholar]
American Nurses Association [ANA]

Real Talk

5-minute writing prompt:
    What are some of the things they didn't tell you about in nursing school that you wish you had known?

Reality Check

While nursing school does a great job preparing us for the transactional foundations of nursing, none of us are prepared for the emotional sh*t show that we will experience. Coupled with unhealed drama and trauma, the unchecked emotions of this profession left me feeling overwhelmed, anxious, co-dependent, burned-out, and alone. I have several coaching tools, videos, and resources that I am happy to share for free if you are willing to raise your hand to become your own solution.

Take Action

Join us in the Facebook community and be a part of the conversation! What do you know now that you wish you had learned in nursing school?
    Follow me on social media for tips, stories, inspiration, and recipes.
    Let's connect! Schedule a call with me.
    Share this book with all the nurses you know. The vulnerable shares, real talk, and tools provided in this book may just save a life.

Scan QR code for more

https://linktr.ee/jessicasmithdossantos

THE SET UP: ALTRUISM, EMOTIONAL COMPOSURE & EMOTIONAL ENDURANCE

W e don't know it, but we are set up for failure from the very beginning. We come to this profession with the secret ingredients for burnout already entangled in our nature. Our altruistic hearts are excited to serve and have not yet been taught the boundaries of giving. Coupled with the superhuman skills of emotional composure and emotional endurance that develop naturally in response to the demands of our profession, it is the making of a perfect storm.

Altruism

Altruism is a general theme of giving to others at the expense of one's self and is universally interwoven into the fabric of human nature. The media has done an excellent job of portraying nurses as superheroes, wearing scrubs and capes. This image implies that we are to be trusted, that we will fight for our patients in their moments of need, and we will stop at nothing to save a life.

The kink of altruistic behavior is that there are rewards. Sherrie Bourg Carter, Psy.D writes in her article for Psychology Today that the rewards of altruism include: a helper's high from the release of endorphins, increased feelings of satisfaction and gratitude, improved physical health, and even distraction from personal problems. The challenge with altruism is that the high of the reward camouflages the signs of burnout until it is too late.

Clear! Everybody Clear!

It was Valentine's Day. I remember, because there was a huge bowl of candy grams at that charge desk that we could purchase and pass on to a co-worker. Just a little festive fun for those of us who were working the day away.

I needed to pee and was thinking about what I was going to eat for lunch and who I would like to send a candy gram to when I received a call from the lobby informing me that I had been assigned a new patient and I needed to come get him STAT.

"I guess I'll hold it," I thought to myself, trying to forget about my bladder. The thought of making a quick stop at the bathroom on my way to get a patient had not crossed my mind.

The second I walked into the triage room, I knew the situation was critical. Sitting in a wheelchair was a large, portly man with a balding head. His cheeks were gray and beads of perspiration dripped down his face.

I could smell his sweat from the doorway. It smelled like fear. His eyes were wide and worried, yet, he looked exhausted.

The hairs on the back of my neck stood at full attention as I drank him in.

The notes indicated he was feeling light-headed and his blood pressure was low, but there was something else wrong with this picture.

My pulse quickened with a sense of urgency and I made brisk work of getting him back to the room, all thoughts of bathroom breaks, lunch, and candy grams erased from my mind.

I called the tech to assist me in trading his sweat-soaked shirt for a hospital gown and transferring him onto the gurney. I grabbed the heart monitor leads and wiped his wet skin with gauze so it was dry enough for the pads to stick. As soon as a rhythm came onto the screen, all the wrong was righted.

This man was in full ventricular tachycardia. Awake and alert, but the next question was, "for how much longer?"

I had seen it one other time in my career. A patient conscious and talking, but in ventricular tachycardia. It amazed me then and it continues to amaze me now that a human could tolerate such a wild heart rhythm.

I looked at the tech and nodded while simultaneously sticking my head out into the hallway and asking another nurse passing by to grab the crash cart and the ER Doc STAT.

The tech was already opening the supply cart, preparing supplies to start an IV. I anticipated that we would need to defibrillate him in the very near future. I kept calm and started engaging the patient in some light conversation about his symptoms while pulling on gloves in case I needed to start CPR.

"When did your symptoms start?"

"What were you doing when they started?"

"Have you ever felt this way before?"

The nurse and a second tech came in with the crash cart. One look at the bedside monitor and they snapped into fast action, working in unison to apply the defibrillation pads to the patient's chest wall.

I let the patient know that his heart was in an irregular rhythm and that we would be getting the Doctor in to see him as soon as possible. We were a team in flow. Our training informed our actions and our teamwork informed our roles.

In perfect rhythm with one another, the IV was established with fluids flowing, the defibrillation pads were in place. We all took a unified inhale as the patient let out a moan and lost consciousness.

All eyes on me, I flipped on the defibrillator power and hit the "charge" button while calling out, "Clear! Everybody clear!"

One last inspection to ensure the safety of my teammates and I called out "Shock!" while pushing the defibrillate button, delivering 120 joules of electricity to the patient's heart. His body jolted off the bed and we all looked with anticipation from the monitor to the patient and back to the monitor, expert hands posed to start chest compressions. To our collective relief, the monitor showed that the cardioversion had successfully converted him back to a normal sinus rhythm and the patient was already regaining consciousness.

That was when it came to our awareness that the ER physician had been standing in the doorway of the room, observing the action. The patient looked at him and smiled, "I feel so much better!"

"I bet you do," replied the ER Doc. He looked at me and said, "Well, I guess you don't really need me anymore!"

We all let out a laugh. I suppose he was right. We had literally brought a man back from the dead on Valentine's Day! Once the patient was stable, I excused myself to the bathroom as my bladder had started cramping in protest.

Later that day, there was a candy gram on the desk in my workstation. It read, "Thanks for saving my life. From, your Patient".

Damn that felt good. The glory, the recognition, the badass Superhero Nurse and her team just saving lives![2]

---

[2] **Source:**
Bourg Carter, S (2014). Helper's High: The Benefits (and Risks) of Altruism [Psychology Today]

Real Talk

5-minute writing prompt:
When was a time in your career when you felt like a hero?

Reality Check

"A hero is someone who voluntarily walks into the unknown."
—Tom Hanks. Every shift, every patient, every interaction is an unknown for a nurse. We are tasked to care for strangers with symptoms that could go sideways at any moment.

Take Action

Join us in the Sh*t They Don't Tell You in Nursing School community and tell us your hero story!

Scan QR code to join

https://linktr.ee/jessicasmithdossantos

Obviously, in matters of life and death, impending death trumps all else. My bladder and my hungry tummy may have suffered a little, but altruism saved a life that day. That's how it starts. One life was saved. One good high as a reward for letting my bladder cramp and my belly stay hungry. One sugary prize for a job well done. The price of personal discomfort was eagerly paid for the life of another.

Altruism is the gateway drug to more and more sacrifice.

Without awareness and boundaries, altruism starts to bleed slowly and insidiously into the makeup of our personalities. We start mistaking the trait of altruism for WHO WE ARE.

It would seem that we are programmed, over time, to believe that altruistic selflessness and self-sacrifice are just part of our identities as nurses. We are rewarded for our sacrifice, enticed with free food and extra pay, and praised for showing up again and again for overtime.

We buy into the superhero persona because it strokes the Ego. We can always justify not caring for ourselves if it means that someone else is being cared for. Our altruistic nature blurs the lines of our boundaries—both personally and professionally—and we find ourselves saying "yes" to way too much.

We chronically overcommit ourselves, no matter how exhausted we become. Like a baby elephant with a ball and chain on our ankles, we keep doing what we have always done. We embrace the discomfort. We keep showing up. We provide. We give. We become desensitized to the burden and blind to the cost.

Like that baby elephant, altruism becomes the weight that makes us believe there is no way to freedom because we have always been trapped.

Didn't Want to, But Did

I sat up in bed, snuggled in my blanket with my morning cup of tea; my hair a lion's mane of bedhead mess. I was groggy from a restless night, too awake to go back to sleep, but too sleepy to be up and about.

I smiled at the sound of the house waking up, the pitter patter of little feet outside my bedroom door. I could hear their dad whispering, "Shhh. Mom's sleeping," as he attempted to shoo them down the hall. I was grateful to have some space to just be; no one needed anything from me, no thoughts in my head. Just quiet bliss. It was a rare peaceful moment in a hectic ER nurse, busy momma, wife kinda life.

My body sank back against the pillows, soft and fluffy, embracing my tired body in a warm hug. It felt so good to just do nothing. I let my neck roll around in gentle circles, exploring the full range of relaxed motion, my shoulders softening.

As I exhaled, a soft, "Mmmmmm," escaped my lips. I was enjoying being fully present with the tender stretches. My head lolled back on the pillow, as my eyelids drooped closed over my tired eyes.

I inhaled; the scent of warm apples and cinnamon wafting out of my tea cup guided me into a memory of baking apple pies with my children. I smiled as I envisioned my daughter, still an infant, propped up on the counter in her light teal Bumbo chair waving the spatula around in the air. Her little cheeks were rosy from teething, drool dribbling down her chin.

My son stood on a chair next to me. His bare feet pranced excitedly, his diaper hanging from his little hips, his naked chest quivering with excitement as I let him dip the measuring spoon into the bag of sugar and sprinkle it over the top of the freshly cut apples.

My heart softened and a happy tear escaped the corner of my eye. There had not been a lot of happy memories with my babies lately. They were now 4 and 6, and we were going through a rough time. I was barely keeping it together trying to figure out how to pay our mountain of bills, work full-time, navigate marriage, process the chaos of work in the ER, take care of 3 dogs and 2 little ones, and still have the energy to do fun things. I had turned into an exhausted, short tempered, "let's watch another movie" mom.

Happy tears turned into sad ones as my thoughts wandered to my current reality. I allowed myself to cry. To feel the sadness in my chest and to let the hot tears flow. It had been a long time since I had the space and the privacy to reveal all of myself and to let my sad out.

My phone, sitting face down next to me on the night stand, began to vibrate. I sighed, sniffed my drippy nose, and lifted up the phone. Looking at the screen through tear-blurred eyes, I recognized the number from work.

Of course. They need me.

I sat there, warm tea in one hand, vibrating phone in the other, and felt the muscles in my neck and shoulders tighten while the peanut gallery in my head started debating.

"Answer it!" One voice said.

"It is obviously important if they are calling you on your day off!"

"Don't do it!" Said another. "This is your day off. You are so exhausted. You need to stay home and take care of yourself."

"But it has to be super important," chimed in yet another. "You know they need your help. You heard them talking at the charge desk yesterday, they are so short staffed. You know you are such a good nurse and you add so much value to the team!"

"Shut up! Both of you," the second voice said. "Don't listen to any of that noise. They have already taken enough of your heart, your soul, your time, and your energy. You don't owe them anything. Their short staffing problem is not yours to solve."

The phone stopped vibrating and I sighed in relief. Inaction had silenced the debate and it was back to me and my cozy blanket. I set the phone back on the nightstand, facedown. I dragged in a long deep breath of air and let it out slowly, feeling the tension of the momentary debate dissipate from my neck and shoulders.

No sooner had I sunk back into the pillows when the phone vibrated again. This time, a text.

"Don't even think about it!" Voice 2 started up again. "Turn that thing off and rest. You need this time! You deserve it!"

The other 2 voices joined in, united, "You know you have to look! You can't not look. If you don't look, you won't be able to enjoy this moment anyway! Your mind will just sit here wondering what the text is about! Just look at it!"

"Ugh!" I groaned, reaching for the phone again. I turned it over and glanced at the screen.

"Staff needed ASAP for day and night shift. Call charge." The SOS notification for help gleamed back at me. The mental debate began again.

"Get up, get dressed. Let them know you are coming in. Your kids will be fine with their dad today. He won't complain about you going in to work extra. You know you need the money," said Voice 1.

"Yea!" said Voice 3. "Get up! You know they need you at work. They always need you. Think about your poor co-workers, short staffed and slammed. They come in to help you. You should go in to help them. They need you!"

"Exactly! They need you! Come on! You can rally and make it happen. Just get up and get moving," Voice 1 added.

The thoughts came in so hard and so fast. If I didn't go, my co-workers would drown with all the work. No breaks, no help, and slammed with an unsafe patient to staff ratio.

If I don't go, that ONE patient might have to wait too long in the lobby and could die. If I don't go, someone could make an error because they are stretched too thin and rushing. If I don't go, no one else is going to come in the next time I am slammed at work and in need of extra hands. If I don't give, I don't get.

I sighed and leaned forward, uncrossing my legs, and set my bare feet on the floor, preparing to respond to the call for help.

"Are you kidding me?!" Voice 2 hopped in angrily. "You are exhausted right now; you have ONE DAY OFF. ONE DAY. And you want to give that up, too? You are supposed to be having a much-needed family day! How much more can you give to that place before your whole life falls apart?"

I had to admit, that was a valid point. I leaned back against the pillows.

"If you hadn't seen that call or looked at that text, what would you be doing right now?" Voice 2 asked.

I sat in silence for a minute and pondered that question. Truth be told, I would probably be relaxing on my bed, thinking through my life challenges, crying some much-needed tears—and maybe, if I was lucky, I would get a little nap, snuggled with my babies.

I let my head sink into the plush pile of pillows again. That option sounded really good. Exactly what I needed, actually. I needed rest. I needed time to be sad. I needed to just be with me, to be with my family—no endless flood of patients needing care. Just time to be.

I wrangled with the decision to stay home and take care of myself and enjoy time with my family or to go in and serve the community and my co-workers and make some extra cash. I didn't want to go. I wanted to stay home and just check out for a while.

"Damn it! Why didn't I just turn my phone off?" I slammed my head back into the headboard as I let out an exasperated sigh.

I was having such a rare, beautiful moment with myself. Thinking, reflecting, relaxing, enjoying tea, and the peace of the morning. Now, my mind was a shit storm of chatter. My shoulders had become earrings again; my once relaxed muscles were knotted and tense. I sighed, massaging my stiff shoulders with my free hand.

"I am so tired," I thought. "UGH! I am calling them back and telling them I am coming in. I have one set of scrubs in the laundry basket that aren't too bad; I can wear those again."

I hadn't done laundry in over a week. I was so behind in my life!

I stood up from my bed and my blanket fell to the floor. I stepped over it, leaving it in a soft, fluffy heap, and walked to the bathroom. I eyeballed the mound of dirty laundry flowing over the laundry bin and shook my head in disapproval.

"What am I doing with my life?" I wonder. "Here I am, ditching out on myself and my kids for work. They need me and we need the money."

Tears pushed from the back of my eyes and I angrily brushed them away. I felt so empty, so heavy, so sad...

I didn't want to go, but truth be told, I didn't really want to stay, either. Forcing myself to be positive and loving when my marriage had become awkward, was too difficult.

Working so hard to muster up a smile and the patience to sit and play with my children sounded even more exhausting than a 12-hour ER shift.

——————————————————————

My heart hurt. I felt like a terrible
mother and wife because I didn't have
anything left to give to the ones that
were the most important to me.

My heart hurt. I felt like a terrible mother and wife because I didn't have anything left to give to the ones that were the most important to me.

Even with that hurt, my altruistic Superhero Nurse persona kept pulling my focus back to work. I knew that my co-workers were feeling the strain of burnout just as much as I was and I also knew that having extra hands to serve our patients made a difference.

I justified my decision to go to work by thinking about our financial goals. The extra cash helped us to pay off debt. Looking back, if I am really being honest, going to work to save lives felt better than being home in a sinking ship that I felt helpless to save. It was a selfless and sacrificing act just as much as it was a selfish one.

My thoughts turned to the SOS call for help at work. "I don't have a choice. Work needs me. There's no one else. No one else but me." I thought.

I saw the blood on the floor of the ER. I saw the new nurse I met yesterday in my mind. Her face flashed before me as I remembered that panicked look in her eyes. I knew she would be at work today.

She needs me. She can't do this by herself. My kids are little and they will be fine with their dad.

I stood there in the bathroom, my bare feet on the cool tile floor. The dirt grinding up into my naked soles. I felt so pulled in all these directions. What should I do? Work needs me. My kids need me. I need me. I'm supposed to....

Hell, I'm supposed to be better than this. I'm a fucking mess.

Again, the tears threatened to well up behind my eyes. "No! Not today!"

My spine stiffened and the muscles in my upper back tensed as I shook off the weakness and found my strength. My hands turned into a fist around my mug and I slammed it down on the counter with such force that tea sloshed over the sides, and the ceramic handle broke off.

"AHHHHH!!!" I screamed at the ceiling. I tossed the handle carelessly into the sink as I glanced at the puddle of tea on the counter and shrugged. *Whatever.*

I walked back over to the bed and sent my husband a text, as tears started to flow out of my eyes. "Hey. I am needed at work today and I know we could use the money. I'm getting ready to leave."

I wasn't blind to the fact that my babies were growing up without me and my marriage was slowly falling apart; but saving lives in the ER took priority.

Going Home

At some point, altruism will fail.

Home used to be my safe place; the one place I would come back to after a hard day and to relax and check in to the things that brought me joy.

But that stopped being true for me. I had neglected my home and given so much to my profession; my home was falling apart. It had become just one more place where people needed from me that I couldn't give. My cup had run empty.

It was a particularly difficult day at work. Lots of traumas, too many deaths, and a lobby full of rude, entitled, demanding patients.

My sweaty scrubs stuck to my back as I fell into the seat of my car. I felt dirty and used. You know that scene in the Disney movie Hercules where he goes into the underworld to save Meg? As he swims though the sea of souls, they grab onto him, pull at him, grasp at any piece they could get ahold of.

As he continued to swim, you could see life being drained from him. His muscles became weak, the color drained from his face, his skin turned ashen gray. His being became haunted, ghastly, and shriveled.

He kicked and clawed through the souls with the single desperate focus of saving Meg. His very life was being siphoned away, consumed by the eternally parched souls of the underworld; desperate to consume every drop of his being. With every kick, every claw to reach her, he becomes more dead.

That was what I felt like. Hollow. Shriveled. Ghastly. The patients clawing, grabbing, gripping, pulling, sucking away every ounce of my being in their own desperation.

I looked at myself in the rearview mirror and a haggard shell of a person stared back at me.

My gloomy eyes were empty and lifeless, framed by dark circles. My greasy hair stuck to my forehead. My lips were chapped from dehydration. My stomach shrunken from lack of food. It was as if, like Hercules, I had tried to swim down into the endless sea of souls to do a good deed and was left just as dead and desperate as the rest of them.

At least Hercules was given immortality so he could finish the job. I was not so lucky. I was told to go home and rest up because we were short staffed tomorrow. Fuck.

My weary neck went limp and my head hit the headrest. I still had to drive home to where my children would need cuddles and my husband would need sex. I just couldn't. My face wrinkled into an ugly cry face and hot tears started rolling down my cheeks at the idea of having to give more of myself. I considered calling home and telling him that I had to work overtime so I could just sit in my car for a few hours.

If I waited long enough, everyone would be asleep by the time I got home and I could sneak in quietly so as not to wake them. Like a thief slinking through the house, I could go unnoticed. No one wanting hugs. No one needing my attention. I could be at peace with myself and not have to give them what they wanted from me. There was nothing left.

A sob escaped my throat. My heart ached. My skin crawled, thinking about my kids rushing me, their little hands outstretched, excitedly needing the feeling of my skin on theirs. I didn't want to be touched. Couldn't bear to be touched by the people I loved; by the children I dreamed of having. I couldn't go to the place that used to fill my cup and revive my soul.

There was no way they could possibly understand how I felt. This was so unfair to them. So unfair to me. It was like that song "Closing Time" by Semisonic. "Closing time, you don't have to go home, but you can't stay here."

I picked up the phone and called home.

"Hey," I said. "It has been a really gross day and my clothes are definitely contaminated. I will need your help keeping the kids distracted so I can sneak in, strip down, and go straight to the shower."

"No problem," he said. Our interactions had become sterile. I knew he was not getting what he needed from the marriage and I was overwhelmed and incapable of giving.

I hung up the phone and sighed a heavy sigh. At least I had bought myself enough time to have some peace in the shower.

Maybe I could get my mind right and be open to the kids cuddling before bed. Maybe the hot water would wash away the feeling of hands pulling at me and I would be able to tolerate being touched a little more today. No way was I having sex. Absolutely not. Maybe snuggles. Definitely no sex.

Altruism bred feelings of confinement, resentment, and anger. Rather than focusing on all the ways I had created my situation, I made the profession of nursing the villain of my story and the cause of my suffering.

It took me way too long to pull my head out of my ass and realize that feeling oppressed in my life and subordinating to my altruistic, self-sacrificing nature was not an everyone and everything else problem, it was a ME PROBLEM!

It took me way too long to pull my head out of my ass and realize that feeling oppressed by a struggling system and subordinating to my altruistic, self-sacrificing nature was not an everyone and everything else problem; it was a ME PROBLEM!

I was not a prisoner of my employer or my profession. I was not oppressed by the bills that I agreed to pay. I was not a victim of marriage or of motherhood. My PERSPECTIVE was. I was the only one keeping myself trapped. The truth was, I was looking outside of myself for a solution to feel better and when none of those outside resources had an answer to save me, I gave up. I drank alcohol, gorged on chocolate, cried in the shower and binge ate to numb my despair. Altruism had me trapped in a prison of victimhood.

What finally saved me from myself was the willingness to take full responsibility for my experience and decide that I was the only one making me feel any kind of way. I learned to lovingly say no. I leaned into getting in touch with myself and aligned my commitments to the things I most valued. I began to prioritize my own health and well-being. I took the time to understand where the giving boundary was for myself. I chose to focus on what I directly controlled and let the rest go. I became more selfish.

Real Talk

5-minute writing prompt:
In what ways has the profession of Nursing been the villain of your story?

Reality Check

The chaos created by unchecked altruism serves to wake you up to YOU! Pay attention to your language. Let "have to", "need to", and "should" be your cues to take a closer look at why you are agreeing to do what you are doing. One of my favorite quotes is, "'No' is a complete sentence." Each time you say 'no' to one thing, you automatically say 'yes' to something else—make sure it's something you value; something that steers you forward on the path to who you were created to be.

Take Action

Join us in the S**t They Don't Tell You in Nursing School community and share with us your thoughts about altruism and how it relates to the profession of Nursing.

Scan QR code to join

https://linktr.ee/jessicasmithdossantos

Altruistic to the Core

During the writing process with my writing coach, Isabel Lerma, I found myself struggling with this section. Instead of using our usual strategies of 5-minute writing prompts, stories, or letters, I had the opportunity to tap into my inner poet. This poem came first, and the rest of the section flowed from here. Enjoy!

Altruistic to the core
We put the needs of all others before

Ourselves because when we do
In our hearts we feel most true

Disinterested and selfless concern for others
The Fathers, the Mothers, the Sisters, the Brothers

Altruistic to the core
Our own health and well-being we ignore

Self-sacrifice at its most fine
To rest, to nourish, to recharge, we decline

We keep pushing, running, moving to the next
Our Superhero Nurse muscles flexed

Altruistic to the core
Out of our empty cup we continue to pour

For those that are thirsty will never stop
Even when we are down to our last drop

Is there a price that we will pay?
What happens on that day?

Altruistic to the core
What happens on the day we have no more?

No more to give, all used up
Dry to the bone sits our cup

Exhausted, resentful, sick, and burned-out
The price we will pay before our souls will shout,

"Altruistic to the core
This is the day I say NO MORE!

This doesn't work; I've lost myself!
My energy gone, depleted of wealth!"

Our cups run dry, in need of refill
We give and give and give until

Altruistic to the core
Remember what this life is for.

To make memories, enjoy, rest, have fun
For our work here is far from done

Learning to balance our time and treasure
The universe will teach us to take close measure

Altruistic to the core
Put your feet up, relax, restore

Life can end in the blink of an eye
It's not too late, come on, just try

Put yourself first, find balance, yourself revive
For you deserve to live, fully alive.

Altruistic to the core
Your soul is begging you to explore

Only giving from the overflow
Deep down inside, the truth you know.

When you are truly at your best
You keep your cup full and only give from the rest.

Maxi Pad Man

I mentioned that the profession was dynamic. Emotionally heavy, yes. But also, hilarious.

Friends and family often ask me to share stories of when I was a nurse. While the non-medical people in my world have no stomach for what I did as a nurse, they all have a morbid curiosity and ask me to tell stories. This one is a general crowd pleaser: gross enough to be interesting, and funny enough to give a giggle.

I know, it sounds totally wrong: Maxi Pad Man? What the hell?

I hear you, but hang with me. I promise it will be worth your while.

It was a seemingly—dare I say it—QUIET day in the ER. Of course, the second I even thought of the "Q" word, was when it happened.

My eyes took in the scene as the paramedic crew rushed through the door.

A large, grizzly bear of a man lay on his side on the gurney. Legs outstretched, one hand propped under his head, the other on his hip. It was a contradictory scene. A burly dude propped up on his side and posing like a swimsuit model.

I looked at the paramedic with questions flashing in my eyes and in return he broke eye contact and looked down at his feet in a very poor attempt to hold back a laugh. Something devious was afoot.

"Maxi Pad Man has arrived," the patient bellowed.

I jumped, startled in response to the booming, burly voice. The paramedics burst out laughing at what was clearly still an inside joke. I was confused and my nurse Spidey senses told me something was wrong, but I couldn't help but join in the laughter.

I noticed that Maxi Pad Man was sweating; large beads of perspiration formed on his forehead and trickled down the side of his face, as a wet stain started to form on the collar of his shirt. *What the hell am I getting myself into?*

Maxi Pad Man's tiny wife lingered in the doorway. Her petite 5'1" frame was graceful and feminine in a flowing, fall-colored dress; her light brown curly hair pulled up in a messy bun on top of her head. Her frazzled eyes darted to and fro, searching for someone, anyone. She looked scared and frail. I locked eyes with her and gently led her to a chair in the room where she could sit while the tech came to help remove Mr. Maxi's clothes.

The tech reached the part where he was about to remove Mr. Maxi's boxers when the man boomed, "I have an announcement!"

His wife flinched; her lips pressed into a thin, stressed line; her eyes pinched shut. The tech and I stopped dead in our tracks, equally startled. He was a large man with an even larger voice. We looked at each other with wide eyes, not sure we were ready to hear whatever was coming next. Does he need to pee? Is he gonna shart? Was he going to tell us a lame story about how he "slipped" in the shower, magically falling on the shampoo bottle that was now lost up his ass?

Maybe that was why his wife looked so pasty-faced. Poor lady.

"I'm a real man, ok? A real man's man, if you know what I mean."

"Ok, we understand," I replied apprehensively—not really understanding. The tech and I exchanged knowing glances; I would have put money on something being lost up his ass. The tech moved to remove the man's boxers.

"Wait, wait, wait, I think I need to prepare you…"

"Here we go, confession time," I thought to myself.

I looked at the tech again, my eyebrows raised in anticipation. I could see the inner Judgy Bitch in my mind's eye. She had her arms crossed over her chest, hip protruding to the side, red framed readers propped on the edge of her nose. Her hair was pulled back in a tight bun with the air of authority of a librarian about to deliver an ass chewing. "Don't you know by now to always put a string on it? Then you don't end up here, with us removing your pants, embarrassing your poor wife because your asshole sucked it in, causing you to lose all control of the fun. Poor woman." (I told you she was a Judgy Bitch.)

"My hemorrhoid exploded like a postpartum hemorrhage! I'm wearing a Maxi pad! I feel like I just hit puberty and the cramps hurt like hell!"

I laughed out loud; I couldn't help it. We all did. Even his pinched-face wife relaxed a little, a small crack of a smile appearing at the corner of her mouth. My inner Judgy Bitch sat down, crossing one leg over the other. A little disappointed that she was wrong.

I peeled back his shorts as he cahooted in laughter, still sweating, still clenching his fists—obviously in pain. Now, the sweating and the iron metallic twang of blood in the air made a lot of sense. The tech held up his gloved hand, and pinched between his thumb and pointer finger was said maxi pad in all its gory glory.

We exchanged glances again, this time more somber. This was serious. The maxi pad was a large cotton pony and it was completely saturated in blood. Dripping. We both looked at his anus and noted bright red blood flowing pretty heavily. The tech tossed the maxi pad in the trash on his way out the door to get an ER Doctor to the bedside STAT. I eyeballed the IV to be sure it was a large bore and flowing well. This guy was going to crash if we didn't keep his tank full.

"I was gonna put a tampon up there," Maxi Pad Man said, "but I couldn't figure out how to put the damn things in! My wife won't ever stick a finger up there—no matter how many times I ask her."

"Stop it," she squealed, and started to cry. "I can't lose you, Honey. I can't! I just can't! This is not funny right now!"

He looked at her, and his eyes softened. "My angel, of course you won't lose me… but really if I make it through this and come home, will you then stick a finger up there at least one time? Or let me do you?"

"Stop it, you crazy old geezer!" She blushed, but we all giggled. She looked at me, clearly uncomfortable with the conversation.

"It's ok," I reassured her, "people say the craziest stuff in here."

"I bet you guys never had a man's man like me comin' in on his period before! OWWWWWWWW SHITTTT FUCK," Mr. Maxi Pad moaned, as a cramp ripped into his body.

I grabbed a pile of gauze and held firm pressure on his hemorrhoid to try to stop the bleeding while waiting for the ER Doc to arrive.

"Oooooow!" he bellowed.

"I'm sorry. I'm sorry. I have to do it! It may not be a finger, but it is a lot of pressure, my friend!"

"No kidding! You haven't even taken me out for dinner and you are already on third base here!"

I glanced at his wife, trying not to giggle. She rolled her eyes and shook her head from side to side, as a slight smile danced on her lips.

He looked over at his wife, "I think you should know, I have changed my mind, Babe. I don't want you to put your finger up my ass!"

We all chuckled and looked at each other. As messed up as the whole scene was, we were all grateful to have some comedic relief, even if it was a little on the crude side.

Real Talk

5-minute writing prompt:

Write about a time in your career when you were grateful to have some comedic relief.

Reality Check

"A good laugh heals a lot of hurts." — Madeleine L'Engle

Take Action

Join us in the Sh*t They Don't Tell You in Nursing School community and share some of your funny and feel-good stories with us.

Scan QR code to join

https://linktr.ee/jessicasmithdossantos

Emotional Composure and Endurance

Emotional composure is a skill that develops organically throughout the course of your nursing career. It goes hand-in-hand with selflessness and compassion. Over time, you gain the ability to remain calm and composed while simultaneously being ripped apart inside by an emotional tornado.

Emotional endurance involves progressively developing the capacity for emotional composure, enabling you to withstand more and for a longer duration than most individuals. Emotional composure looks like:

- Handling 5 call lights going off all at once with patience and grace even though you are feeling overwhelmed, pressured, and have to pee.
- Maintaining your cool when a patient verbally attacks you even though you actually want to throat punch him for being so freaking rude.
- Using your active listening skills when a family member yells in your face about how their parent is the most important priority and they don't feel that they are getting the finest VIP experience the hospital has to offer. Meanwhile, your body is still coursing with adrenaline and soaked in sweat from the code you just finished running (BTW, your patient died and you still have to pee).
- Bearing the burden of the Doctor's bad mood as he or she stomps around the nurse's station barking orders as if those tasks are the only ones on your very full list that need to be completed. Never mind the fact that you are still trying to chart on that code from earlier, still have to pee, and are starting to get hungry.

- Responding to your patient's snark and sarcasm and irritation with a "Yes, sir, I understand your frustration." The fact that you want to scream that it is not your fault that the CT scanner is broken for the THIRD time this week, is never expressed. Service recovery, service recovery, service recovery, and now, the hangry is creeping in and your level of patience is dwindling (Oh! And you STILL have to pee).
- Mustering the courage to answer a call light of a hungry, thirsty, and angry patient whose test results are delayed at least another hour and pressing the call light to complain is the only thing that is helping her pass the time. You know it is unprofessional to tell her you have not eaten or had anything to drink in more hours than she has and you have been holding your urine for way too many hours at this point.
- Maintaining your kindest and most professional nursing face when inside you want to tell all the patients to EFF ALL THE WAY OFF because at this point you are hours beyond hungry, and mostly because of the pain you are feeling from having to hold your pee.

Emotional endurance looks like tolerating all that bullshit over and over 12-hour shift after 12-hour shift until it becomes just another day. You become anesthetized and what was first overwhelming, becomes average and expected. What most people could never tolerate for more than about 20 minutes, we tolerate for days, weeks, months, and years at a time. We normalize the abnormal.

But hey! That's how us nurses roll. We are excellent at putting on our game faces and getting the "sweet nurse" tone just right to appease almost any situation. We have perfected the appearance of emotional composure in the midst of internal turmoil.

It doesn't matter if our patient in the next room just died. Or if we just helped stabilize a baby that was severely physically abused. Or if the patient we just discharged told us to f**k off and threw his discharge paperwork at us. Or if the patient we checked in was drunk and spat in our faces. Every time we have an interaction with a new patient, to them, none of these things matter. The only thing that matters to them is their needs.

We are able to tolerate some of the most difficult, demanding situations one minute, and then walk into the next patient room as if our day has been nothing but snacks, bathroom breaks, and rainbows.

Emotional freaking composure, baby.

Here's the problem with emotional composure the way we have learned. We are not processing any of those emotions in a way that serves us. We are putting on a mask, pretending, and numbing. We are not developing the skill of emotional composure; we are developing a dangerous ability to suppress and repress emotions.

Here's the problem with emotional composure the way we have learned. We are not processing any of those emotions in a way that serves us. We are putting on a mask, pretending, and numbing. We are not developing the skill of emotional composure; we are developing a dangerous ability to suppress and repress emotions.

We are praised for keeping our shit together and are taught how to numb out. Management rewards us with chocolate, doughnuts, pizza, and tacos. We reward ourselves and each other with drinks after work as a way of connecting in our trauma and helping ourselves feel better.

We talk about the details of our crazy shifts and we make light of the circus, but we never actually talk about the shit show going on deep inside. That tornado of fear, anger, guilt, resentment, sadness. Sometimes those feelings are too dynamic to even name, much less process.

We were never taught how to manage emotions in healthy ways that allow for release and healing. We become masters at suppressing our feelings and then disguising them behind an "everything is ok" mask. We never really let anyone fully see behind the curtain and numbing becomes the norm until one day we describe ourselves as depressed, anxious, and burned-out, and apathetic.

Priding ourselves on being able to show extreme emotional composure for long periods of time is one of the biggest mistakes we can make as nurses. When we start adopting these traits as our identity rather than treating them like a skillset, we set ourselves up for emotional chaos in all areas of our lives.

We forget how to set and maintain healthy boundaries. We start tolerating bullshit in our relationships.

Perpetuating the persona of nurses as superheroes discredits the parts of us that are human and feel an immense amount of emotion. Emotional suppression hinders our ability to connect to our emotions properly and has us hiding the truth behind a mask.

We are left suppressing all the feelings until we rob ourselves of feeling all together. Not feeling at all becomes preferable over feeling the crap that we have no skills to be able to navigate.

Welcome to the ER.

Eight years into my nursing career, I had the opportunity to take a day shift position in the level 2 Trauma Center ER. It was not a role that I was actively looking to take, but an opportunity that I could not turn down.

I had worked telemetry for much of my career and was currently employed in a pre and post procedure unit, which was an easy role. We started a lot of IVs and prepped and recovered patients from simple same-day procedures. We did a few cardioversions on the unit and vigilantly watched for post procedure bleeding.

In terms of critical thinking skills, it was low key. I leveraged that season in my career to go back to school and complete my bachelor's degree and make babies. I was very pregnant with my second child and I had ZERO critical care experience when the ER opportunity came my way.

I struggled with a rough pregnancy and my husband at the time was unemployed. The financial burden of our household was on my shoulders and I had just enough paid time banked to take three months of paid maternity leave after my daughter was born. It was a stressful time financially for us and my OB had already threatened bedrest as my blood pressure was borderline too high.

That's when we received the news that we were to have a mandatory staff meeting in which they announced that they were shutting our department down completely. The unit I worked for was closing and that transition was happening inside of a few short weeks.

The HR representative was present during that meeting to check in with each of us as their desire was to retain us as employees of the organization. They asked us where we may be interested in working, and I stupidly said, "I have always thought ER would be fun."

I had an interview that very day with the management in ER and I was hired on the spot and given my choice of which shift I wanted to work. It was kind of a blur.

Very pregnant, I was fired from a cush pre and post procedure unit job, and hired in the ER with no ICU experience on a day shift all in 4 hours' time.

Looking back, an ER hiring a very pregnant me with no critical care experience to a day shift on spot should have been a red flag warning. Why would a level 2 trauma center ER hire a very pregnant nurse with no critical care experience on a day shift?

Truth be told, they had just had a mass exodus of talented staff and were desperate to replace them. I felt grateful to still have a job, but hadn't really connected the dots of what I would be walking into.

I think I lasted two weeks on orientation in the ER before I was put on bedrest at 31 weeks pregnant for preterm contractions. My daughter was born at 33 weeks and weighed 3 lbs. 12 oz. The financial stress at home, coupled with being tossed into an ER— untrained and unprepared—was enough to put my body in crisis. That was only the beginning.

When I returned to the ER after three months maternity leave, I was sleep deprived, my hormones were a wreck, and I was still trying to take regular breaks to pump breast milk for my very tiny baby. Sometimes, I was so exhausted, that I had to fight to keep my eyes open.

During one of my very first shifts back at work, we had a bad trauma: multiple stab wounds. While I was far from being trauma trained, my mentor thought that it was an imperative part of my orientation to observe the work that happens in the trauma bay.

The patient was an unconscious middle-aged female with approximately 17 stab wounds to her face, chest, abdomen, and upper extremities. We were told that her adult son, who was acutely schizophrenic, believed that she was a werewolf. In an attempt to save himself, he viciously attacked her with a kitchen butcher knife, stabbing her repeatedly.

I stood in the corner of the trauma bay, watching. It was a well-choreographed dance. Each team member had a specific task that played part in a greater symphony. I observed the chaotic yet rhythmic work of this team in awe. It was obvious that they were in a flow with one another that I did not yet fully understand.

I watched as the blood leaked profusely out of the piercing wounds all over the woman's body. Her face, her chest, her arms, her abdomen. So many punctures, so much blood. Some of it spilled off the gurney and onto the floor where it became sticky shoe prints as the trauma team pulsed around her; each one working at rapid speeds to start IVs, transfuse blood and fluids, and compress the bleeding holes. The salty, metallic taste of blood permeated my senses.

I watched as the heart monitor lit up. Blood pressure dropping, heart rate dropping, lights flashing, alarms beeping. The stench of blood, sweat, and adrenaline made me a bit uncomfortable. The energy in the room shifted electric as the team realized that they were losing her and skilled hands started chest compressions.

"Get me the sternal saw." the trauma surgeon demanded in an authoritative and confident tone. I stood in the corner thinking, "Sternal saw? Is he seriously going to cut this woman's chest open, right here in the trauma bay?"

A rush of saliva flooded my mouth and my stomach lurched. I had seen the sternal saw used once before, in my clinical rotation in the OR during nursing school. I had the incredible opportunity to witness an open-heart surgery and I remembered how gruesome the sternal saw was. It reminded me of the jig saw my dad used to cut pieces of wood when I was a kid. Blade teeth ripping through raw material, sawdust tainting the air. I had a moment of panic. My heart raced, and I felt tears well up in my eyes. My breath caught in my throat.

Do I really want to witness them cutting open a human chest?

No, I didn't. I wanted to leave. I wanted to run out of the trauma bay and never look back, but my feet were like lead. Too heavy to lift off the floor. The part of me that wanted to run was held steadfast by the other part of me that was gluttonous to witness. My breath became heavy and thick as my consciousness grappled with my conflicting desires. To run. To stay.

I stayed. I watched the surgeon's skilled hands grip the equipment. I startled a bit at the whirring sound of the sternal saw coming to life, the blade humming, hungry to ravage. The sound it made as it cut into her sternum is not one I will ever forget.

The blade buzzed back and forth, and a high-pitched whine sounded from the machine as the teeth hit the resistance of the sternum. A fine powder of bone and human flesh misted the air. My body shuddered, but my eyes greedily searched for an opening so I could get a better view.

That fine mist of fresh bone dust had barely settled when the surgeon expertly placed the metallic sterile fingers of the rib spreader snugly against the ragged edges of the patient's sternal bone. The crank spread her chest cavity wide, exposing all that is supposed to be sacred to the outside.

He inserted both of his hands into her chest cavity and started manipulating her heart, which was still of all motion—dead in his hands. Cardiac massage, they called it. Warm hands wrapped tenderly, yet desperately, around the muscle of life. I was captivated witnessing the gruesome, yet inspiring, scene of extreme life saving measures.

I walked to the break room, feeling numb and overwhelmed. Her heart had been fatally punctured twice in the left ventricle. She died, brutally stabbed to death by her own son. Her lifeless, naked body lay limp and mutilated on the cold metal of the trauma table; her heart in the surgeon's hands. Some things can never be unseen.

Why did I stay for that?

My legs felt weak and shaky. My stomach turned flips.

"Did I really just get hired into the ER?" I thought as I looked down at my shaking hands.

I sat down on the couch in the break room, and started pumping breast milk for my brand-new baby, and began to sob. The smell of blood, sweat, and adrenaline lingered in my nostrils. The shock of the violence that one human could inflict on another settled into my fragile and innocent soul. The sound of the sternal saw—now probably silent and sterile—still reverberated in my ears as tears flowed down my cheeks.

Welcome to the ER.

I had not yet developed the level of emotional composure or endurance necessary to navigate this new role. Honestly, I think I cried almost every shift for my first year. If I didn't cry in the bathroom or the breakroom, I definitely cried on my drive home.

That was when I was still in touch with what I was feeling and allowed myself the process of expressing the way I needed to. I had at least three meetings with HR in those first six months, begging to be transferred somewhere else—anywhere else.

When they started cross-training me for the pediatric ER, I began feeling more confident. For the most part, it was softer than the adult ER. The pediatric traumas were handled in the trauma bays and the codes were few and far between. With time, I became more assured that I may actually be able to handle being an ER nurse.

My first year in the ER toughened me up. I developed a protective shell. I didn't feel the pain as deeply, I cried less, and I was able to float back to the adult ER to help out. I had stopped contacting HR to change jobs.

Over the course of the next several years, I transitioned back to working mostly in the adult ER. With a lot of exposure to drama and trauma, I developed emotional composure and endurance.

Crying at work was no longer a thing and I took it as a good sign that I was doing great, being strong, settling in. What I didn't know then that I do know now, is that I was not developing the skills of emotional composure and endurance; I was sliding into a protective mechanism.

My lack of tears didn't mean that I was stronger and more capable; it meant that I was detaching from the pain by numbing myself with food and alcohol, and building a wall around myself.

I was learning how to suppress and numb my emotions so that I didn't have to feel.

Numb

Emotional suppression can only be sustained for so long before it starts killing your soul and robbing you of fulfillment.

I reached a point in my career where I realized that I had stopped feeling the bad stuff; the fear, the pain, the shame, the guilt, the resentment, the disgust, and the sadness. At first, I welcomed the numbness. It was such a relief to NOT FEEL all of that crap. Unfortunately, it took me a while to realize that being numb also robbed me of the ability to feel the good stuff too: love, joy, hope, fulfillment, happiness, excitement, connection. I was numb and disinterested, apathetic and withdrawn, burned-out beyond recognition.

I had become a checked-out shell of a woman who showed up, did my job, and went home—didn't really give a shit about anything. I had stopped engaging with my life and it had stopped engaging with me. Like a neglected house plant, all the things I cared so much about were withering away from lack of attention and nourishment.

My relationship with my children suffered. I had become the "let's watch another movie" mom who just wanted to lay on the couch and not have to engage with my kids. I didn't want to go to the park, I didn't want to play games, I didn't want to go outside. I barely wanted to be snuggled. My children overwhelmed me and I didn't enjoy the experience of being a mom.

My bank account suffered. My finances were falling apart around me. We had become trapped in the American Dream. With more debt than we knew what to do with, minimum payments lay claim to every paycheck we brought home. We used credit cards to buy gas and groceries, making the hole deeper and more oppressive each month. Eventually, we were forced to short sell our beautiful, custom built "forever home", leaving our credit score dead in the gutter.

My marriage suffered. After 14 years together, we were separated and navigating heartache, shared custody, and legal paperwork. Splitting assets and squabbling over things. Deciding who would have the kids and when.

Truth be told, letting my marriage fall apart provided a sense of relief. Relief that I wouldn't have to come home and face the disappointment on his face when I was not interested in interacting. Relieved that I didn't have to explain myself anymore. Relieved that I didn't have one more person who needed something from me that I couldn't and didn't want to give.

My physical health suffered. I carried around 65 extra pounds. My skin was broken out like a teenager from all the crap I consumed. My joints ached and I had no energy. I could sleep for 10 hours solid and still not feel rested. I struggled to stay awake. I felt like it was all I could do to drag myself through the day. I medicated with sugar and caffeine in an attempt to keep myself awake, destroying my health even further in the process.

My mental health suffered. I was numb. Swindled out of the rich tapestry of emotion which adds depth and memory to this human experience. I was trapped in my own existence. Defeated, resigned to the reality of "the way things were", with little hope of change.

My self-image suffered. I didn't recognize the woman looking back at me in the mirror. She was haggard. She had dark bags under her eyes and puffy swollen cheeks. She looked sad and bitter. Her sparkle for life was dead. The woman that was once so excited to create her life, get married, have children, and feel joyful and vibrant was but a memory, tainted by the harsh reality of nursing. The only thing she looked forward to was sleep.

My friendships suffered. Most of the time, I didn't feel like socializing. I didn't want the stimulation of being around people, and I didn't want to put myself in a situation where someone might need something from me when I couldn't even give it to myself. I was so depleted that I was incapable of giving or receiving friendship.

If you know me now, it would be really hard for you to picture me as the woman I just described. I am naturally extroverted. I talk to strangers all the time and most of the time I share a hug before moving on.

I am 41 now and my daughter kindly pointed out the grooves etched in the skin around my face are starting to become permanent evidence of how much I smile every day.

Looking back on that season of my life, I see now that I was so emotionally traumatized, my only option was system shutdown.

Every emotion that is left suppressed just sits there, waiting for the next trigger so it can recycle itself and gain momentum.

That is precisely what leads to burnout both in our personal and our professional lives. The ability to suppress emotion on a superhuman level, creates an inauthenticity within ourselves and we begin to question our own identity and self-worth.

Phrases like "moral injury" and "compassion fatigue" start entering our vocabulary and resentment begins to brew. We are set up from the get go; we are praised for being strong, rewarded for doing it over and over again, and left to figure it out on our own when we find the ashes of our lives scattered around our feet.

The Linen Room

I was hiding in the linen room, sobbing. The tidy, sterile stacks of linens kept me company while I fell apart. My shoulders stiffened when my co-worker came in and caught sight of me.

"Woah, what's up?"

"I'm exhausted. This job is killing my soul and my life. I give so much to everyone and everything that my life is falling apart. My husband moved out over the weekend."

I was so defeated that I couldn't even make the effort to wipe the snot rocket off my upper lip, much less be bothered by the black trails of wet mascara sliding down my face. There I stood, in the height of my ugly cry face glory, looking at him.

He stood there, staring back at me, looking a little shocked and not sure what to say.

We were in similar stages of life. Spouses, small kids, homeowners. We had shared many conversations about the challenges of marriage and the traumas of the job. We had talked about the exhaustion and how it made it hard to care for the little ones after a long day. We had shared concerns for the sustainability of, well, all of it really. I can imagine his marriage flashed through his mind at that moment. Things had been rocky between them as well.

He walked forward and wrapped me in a hug. A little squeak escaped my mouth and more tears came. My face pressed up against his chest, hot tears continued to roll out of my eyes.

When I became a nurse, I thought I had found my forever career. When I married my husband, I thought it was going to be just like the vows; until death do us part.

I didn't invest all of that time and money just to flush a career down the toilet. I didn't say "I do" and work to build 14 years of life together just to tear it all down. I didn't create my beautiful children with the intention of ripping the family apart and putting them through a childhood of separation and divorce.

I hated seeing my son crying because he missed his dad. His heartbreak replayed in my mind and my soul felt like it was being ripped into pieces. I worked so hard to become a nurse and to save people's lives and yet, the ones that mattered the most to me, including my own, were disintegrating. As I stood there, my face buried in my colleague's chest, indulging in my emotions, my mind ran wild.

How did this happen?

How did things get so far gone?

Selfless, altruistic nurse had become my identity. My self-sacrificing behavior had created chaos in my relationships and my finances. Ungoverned altruism birthed burnout in my physical and mental health. My heart felt mutilated. My ability to maintain emotional composure pushed past what I was capable of enduring.

Selfless, altruistic nurse had become my identity. My self-sacrificing behavior had created chaos in my relationships and my finances. Ungoverned altruism birthed burnout in my physical and mental health. My heart felt mutilated. My ability to maintain emotional composure pushed past what I was capable of enduring.

Suddenly, I remembered that I was at work. I inhaled deeply as my mouth took in the fabric of his scrubs, the smell of fabric softener contradicting the sanitary starch of the linen room. As good as it felt to fall apart for a minute, I knew that the remainder of a 12-hour shift was still waiting for me on the other side of the linen room door. As grateful as I was for the comfort of being wrapped in his arms, I knew I needed to get my shit together.

I pushed away from him; my eyes cast down in shame. "Thanks," I whispered as I let myself out.

———————

Altruism, emotional endurance, and emotional composure: the perfect storm. Set up from the beginning to fail, our altruistic hearts were excited to serve, but had not yet been taught the boundaries of giving.

We learn through the feedback of chaos and defeat. And, when we find the ashes of our lives scattered around our feet, hopefully, we make a choice to rise up.

Real Talk

5-minute writing prompt:
   Write about a time when you or someone you know suffered from burnout.

Reality Check

In the numb season of my life, I didn't know what I didn't know. I had no skills to navigate the emotions I felt and checking out was my protection. Emotional numbness was the one state of being that allowed me to be a little bit ok. If that is you right now, I want you to know that you are not alone. There is no judgment, criticism, or expectation in this space. You matter, you are worthy of wholeness, and it is safe to be vulnerable here.

Take Action

Being vulnerable about emotional numbness and burnout can be scary. The first coaching session with me is always free, so let's talk. I'm here for you!

Scan QR code to schedule

https://linktr.ee/jessicasmithdossantos

THE EMOTIONAL SHIT SHOW

Trigger warning: this content may cause some intense emotions. If you are concerned about being triggered, refer to the PAUSE THE HUSTLE section now and at any time throughout this book.

I know that the root of the majority of my suffering as a nurse was never having been taught how to govern my emotions. Fear, shame, guilt, and resentment dominated my experience.

As basic as it seems, there were times when I couldn't even put a label on what I was feeling. Sometimes there were so many emotions all at once that it felt like I was trapped in my own internal tornado with alcohol and chocolate as my only strategy to make it stop. The persona of the nurse as an everyday hero—strong and confident, wearing a cape and celebrated for the sacrifice—became an image that I subordinated my identity to. A persona that leaves no room for feeling feelings.

The community doesn't need to know that our souls are dying a slow death or that we are losing ourselves to the emotional game. We can't afford for our patients to know that we are hurting, second-guessing ourselves, or numbing with drugs or alcohol just to sleep. So, we suffer in silence.

It is lonely, confusing, and overwhelming. Trying to sort out what we have seen and done, trying to process what we didn't do or could have done better. Feeling trapped in our own minds and not sure how to get out.

We are supposed to be strong. We are supposed to be comforting and intelligent. We are supposed to be kind and patient. We are supposed to be advocates and caregivers. We are innately trusted by most and are supposed to be the face, the hands, and the heart of patient care. We are supposed to have strong spines and open hearts. We are supposed to work long hours while short staffed, show up for mandatory overtime, and serve the organization at all costs.

For a while, we manage. We show up, we put our strong faces on and do the do. But over time, we lose ourselves. Our physical and mental health start to decline. Anxiety and depression set in. We check out and stop being engaged in our work and in our lives. The message that we don't really matter sets in and mentally checked-out becomes the new normal simply because we don't know any better. We numb and we lie to ourselves about how burned-out we really are.

Fear

I love how Dr. Alok Trivedi defines fear. He describes it as an emotion of the future caused by one of two things: either losing something you hold dear to you, or gaining something you don't want. Dr. Trivedi says, "You can't fear the past, it is impossible. You can only fear something that has yet to come."

Fear: Losing Something You Hold Dear

The Man in 22

When I was a brand-new nurse, still on orientation, I made a medication error that could have caused a patient to have cardiac arrhythmias so severe that he may have needed a temporary pacemaker. It was back in the days before computer charting was a thing and the paper charts were located on medication carts outside the patient's room.

Here was the situation: The patient in 22 was a middle-aged gentleman on a Heparin drip for blood clots in his legs and was transitioning to oral Coumadin the day I was on shift. He was generally fit and his heart rate was on the lower side of normal at baseline. For those of you who may not know, blood clots are treated with medications that prevent clots from forming. Heparin is the IV form and Coumadin is the oral form of medication that thins the blood and helps prevent the existing blood clots from getting bigger.

The patient in 23 was also a generally fit middle-aged gentleman. He was having cardiac arrhythmias and had been stabilized on IV Amiodarone, which is a powerful antiarrhythmic medication designed to help the heart beat normally. That day he was also scheduled to transition off of the IV and onto oral Amiodarone.

Both middle-aged men, both generally fit, both transitioning from an IV medication to an oral medication. The charts for 22 and 23 shared the same desk as the rooms were right next to each other. Can anyone see the beginning of a set up for a medication error to occur?

I had gained sufficient practical experience as a nursing apprentice during my time in nursing school, which gave me the confidence to lower my guard a bit. Consequently, I found myself being more approachable and engaged in conversations with both of those patients that day. I felt less stressed and more relaxed in my role as a nurse and confident about the tasks on my list.

When it came time to administer 23's oral dose of Amiodarone, I did what I always did and started the process of the '5 rights':

1. Right patient: the chart was outside the door of the patient's room, 23, yup!
2. Right medication: I unlocked the medication drawer, opened the chart, checked the written order, double checked that it had been transposed onto the MAR correctly, and then checked the name on the chart just to be extra sure. Yep, still all good.
3. Right dose: All good there. The order matched the MAR, the MAR matched the medication packaging.
4. Right route: Pill form, to be given orally, yes. Coming off of IV Amiodarone and starting oral Amiodarone.
5. Right time: 0900! Let's do this!!

You might be thinking, "OK, so what exactly is the problem here?"

The problem was that the charts were switched and I was looking at the right patient's chart sitting outside the wrong patient's room!

Here is where it all went wrong. I walk into 22 (not 23!) all confident-like, Amiodarone in hand, and I informed the patient that I had his oral medication for him and that he would be getting rid of that IV today. We joked around about how nice it would be to get rid of the "ball and chain" (that was the IV) as he took the medication.

I never asked the patient to verify his name. I never took a second look at the IV bag to make sure it was Amiodarone. If I had, I would have realized that it was Heparin and I was in the wrong room. I never told him the name of the medication I was giving him. I simply said I was giving him his pill to get off the IV. He took me at my word, and swallowed the pill!

When I finally realized that I had given the Amiodarone to the WRONG FREAKING PATIENT, I felt all sorts of things all at once. Hot sweats, cold palms, dizziness, nausea, and a little like I might crap my pants. Realization is one thing; full-on ownership is another.

When I finally realized that I had given the Amiodarone to the WRONG FREAKING PATIENT, I felt all sorts of things all at once. Hot sweats, cold palms, dizziness, nausea, and a little like I might crap my pants. Realization is one thing; full-on ownership is another.

My stomach hit my feet as I went through the checklist of all that was to follow.

I had to confess my error to my mentor, the patient, the physician that was caring for the patient, the pharmacy (so I could get another dose of the medication for the correct patient), and my management team.

I had to write out a full incident report on the whole mess. Ooh! I forgot to mention, the patient's wife was a total and complete nightmare of a woman. The high strung, Type A, lawyer-like, Alpha female kinda nightmare.

My throat went dry as I pictured her verbally slaughtering me, slaying me with her sword of a tongue, leaving my soul for dead when she found out about the error. *Gulp.*

The worst part was that this patient already had a naturally low heart rate and the medication I had just given him was designed to suppress cardiac activity. This meant that he could potentially need a temporary pacemaker when the medication kicked in, as his heart rate could drop dangerously low.

Last little fun fact: the half-life of Amiodarone (or the amount of time it takes for half of the dose of the drug to clear the human system) was 15-142 days. Basically, there was potential for this guy's heart to have problems for up to 142 DAYS because of what I had just done.

Holy Fucking Shit.
Holy Fucking Shit.
Holy Fucking Shit.

I sat down in a chair in the hallway, emotionally terrorized as I imagined what could happen next. I felt the color drain from my face as I sank back against the wall. I was nauseous and my armpits were drenched with sweat. I seriously considered running back into the patient's room and begging him to force himself to throw up to get the pill back out. Yeah, that was a real thought.

Hear me out. In my panic, I really believed that if he barfed it back up then we could just pretend it never happened and move on with our lives. We would not have to worry about his heart for the next ONE HUNDRED AND FORTY-TWO days. I could beg him to not tell his wife so she wouldn't butcher me where I stood.

"Yeah. That was the solution," I thought to myself, leaning forward in the chair. I would march back into that room, barf bag in hand, confess what I had just done, and beg him to stick his fingers down his throat until he vomited it back up.

Perfect. I squared my shoulders and was just about to stand up when my mentor saw me sitting in the chair in the hallway and came down to find out what was up. I slouched back in the chair and started bawling. HUGE tears rolling down my face. The first thing I said was, "Where do I have to go and turn in my badge when I get fired?"

I was certain my nursing career was over before it had even really begun. I had failed one of the most basic principles of medication administration and I had put a patient's life in danger. Someone who trusted me to care for him. Someone who trusted me with his life. I had put him in danger because I did not follow one of the most basic safety practices in nursing.

I could barely breathe. I hyperventilated like a toddler in the throes of a meltdown as I envisioned myself behind bars wearing an orange prison jumpsuit, stripped of my career and my freedom. It took my mentor some time to calm me down, and I was finally able to tell him what I had done. He took it from there.

He called the physician who came and assessed the patient. He let the patient know what had happened, what it meant for him, and what the plan of care was. He called the pharmacy to obtain another dose of Amiodarone for the correct patient. He filled out the incident report. All while I followed him around like a whipped dog, feeling like a negligent derelict. I can still feel the tears well up in my eyes and my heart starts racing a bit as I retell this story.

I was afraid to re-engage. I was afraid my patient would have some serious health problems and need a pacemaker. I was afraid his wife would sue the hospital and then sue me for what I had done. I was afraid I would lose my job. I was afraid my nursing license would be revoked and my career would be over. I was afraid something even worse would happen.

What if he died?

What if I had to go to prison for the rest of my life for murder?

Just like that, in one swallow, I was done. My career and my life were over. I was afraid to touch another patient or administer another medication ever again.

Obviously, that wasn't the end of me or I wouldn't be sitting here writing a book about a 17-year career and being burned to a crisp. But it was certainly the first time I experienced such intense fear of losing something I held dear to me. My patient's life, my job, my nursing license, my liberty.

I think most of us face at least one terrifying mistake in our careers. A lapse in judgment, a protocol not followed, a medical error. While this was the last time I ever gave the wrong patient the wrong medication, it wasn't the last time I made a mistake over the course of my 17 year career.

I think most of us face at least one terrifying mistake in our careers. A lapse in judgment, a protocol not followed, a medical error. While this was the last time I ever gave the wrong patient the wrong medication, it wasn't the last time I made a mistake over the course of my 17 year career.

While the public may see us as everyday superheroes, we are actually just human. Which means that we are also prone to error, just like every other human. We have a heart to serve. A desire for people to heal and get better. We never intend for errors to occur, but they do.

Making an error that may cause harm to a patient that puts your license at risk is easily one of the worst feelings. An emotional shit storm, without a doubt. As with anything, there is always a lesson, a silver lining, a nugget of wisdom, a wakeup call.

First and foremost, I can tell you that I never went into another patient's room without the chart in my hand to double check the patient's identity. My 5 rights were done at the bedside in earshot of the patient and I made sure I had the patient's buy-in before allowing him or her to take the medication. I became an exceptional mentor for nursing students and new graduate nurses because I was intimately aware of how horrible it felt to make an error that could harm a patient by skipping the basics.

I had a very real and very vulnerable story in my back pocket that I could tell with emotion and from experience that would really drive the point home. And I had a conviction to do my very best to save a new nurse from the pain of a medication error.

As a side note, that process became a whole lot easier and more fool proof with the invention of the electronic medical record and the ability to scan the armband and the medication as the primary method of documentation. As long as the patient had the correct information on the armband, the process was safer and more efficient!

If you are a new nurse or a seasoned nurse who may be a little more relaxed in the 5 rights, I hope that my story refreshes your enthusiasm for the process of safe medication administration.

At this point, you are probably wondering what happened to the patient.

We were so lucky. SO.LUCKY. He was the nicest man and extended an undeserved amount of grace. He could tell how atrocious I felt about what had happened and he actually asked if we could keep it a secret from his wife. I suspect he was also afraid that she would eat me alive. He didn't seem worried at all about what had happened and was aware that this error may mean a temporary pacemaker for him.

Over the next 48 hours, he had no signs of bradycardia or concerns that he would have any ill effects from the medication error, and he went home.[3]

---

[3] **Source:**

Robertson, J; Long, L (2018) *Suffering in Silence: Medical Error and its Impact on Health Care Providers https://pubmed.ncbi.nlm.nih.gov/29366616/*

Real Talk

5-minute writing prompt:

Write about a time when you or someone you know made a medical error.

Reality Check

Even though we have an "RN" behind our name, we are still first and foremost, human; which means that we are also fallible. Because of the level of responsibility we carry in our profession, errors bear a greater weight on our mental and emotional health. One source pointed at medical errors as the source of "burnout, lack of concentration, poor work performance, posttraumatic stress disorder, depression, and even suicidality". (Jennifer J Robertson, Brit Long) If you have made a medical error and are feeling heavy in your head and your heart about it, I want you to hear me loud and clear on this one, you are not alone!

Take Action

Join us in the Sh*t They Don't Tell You in Nursing School community for love, laughs, and real talk. You are welcome to share your error stories with us in the group, but please don't feel that you have to. If you are feeling called to schedule a free coaching session, please do so now. I would love to serve you.

Scan QR code for more

https://linktr.ee/jessicasmithdossantos

Fear: Gaining Something You Don't Want

While I will forever be grateful to the man in 22 for being so gracious and for helping me learn a lesson that shaped me into one of the most diligent nurses when it came to medication administration, I can tell you that not all stories that evoke fear end on a high note.

Sue's Husband

It was another crazy busy day in the ER. The kind of day where help was hard to find because everyone was equally slammed. I was working in the acute care pod and I had a 3-room assignment. Two of my rooms had patients already and my last open room was the last open bed in the acute care pod.

This pod was specifically reserved for the sickest of the sick, which is why we were only assigned three patients at a time. The patients that came to these rooms were the ones that were on the brink of death, were actively receiving CPR, or had significant changes in their vital signs, which indicated that a full system crash was right around the corner. For these patients, time was of the essence and their lives depended on everything we did or didn't do.

The overhead page sounded something like this: "REMSA to 11, ETA 2 minutes. ERP to bedside". Basically, that meant that an ambulance was coming in hot and the patient needed an emergency room physician (ERP) to assess the situation STAT because the patient likely already had one foot in the grave.

Fun Fact: "STAT" is short for the latin word "statim", which means "immediately". Yes, I paused my writing to look it up because I always knew it meant RIGHT NOW, but I had never really known why "STAT" specifically. You're welcome!

Back to the story.

I popped into 11 and started a quick scan to make sure all the equipment was in order.

- Suction canister set up and ready with extra tubing and a wall regulator. Check!
- Adult sized ambu bag ready to roll, oxygen flow meter in place and working. Check!
- Supply cart fully stocked with everything needed to start more than one IV and hang fluids. Check!
- Monitor plugged in and turned on. Check!
- Blood pressure cuff, pulse ox, and EKG stickers at the ready. Check!
- Crash cart parked just around the corner and on standby. Check!

While inspecting my physical environment I simultaneously thought about my other two patients.

When was the last time I checked on them?

Were they stable?

Would they need anything from me in the next hour?

Both were stable and waiting on labs and imaging results. They were tucked in and had the TV remote/call button in hand.

Ready to rock. Let's do this.

Even as I write this, I can feel my heart rate increasing, my awareness rising. The ERP and I watched the stretcher come around the corner. We could see a middle-aged male patient in an upright sitting position with a large, red biohazard bag tied around his neck. He was actively vomiting enormous amounts of bright red blood. His wife was trailing behind, looking rattled and haggard.

As we collectively moved him over to the gurney, we received a report. He had a long-standing history of alcoholism, liver cirrhosis, portal hypertension, and ruptured esophageal varices. His wife shared that he continued to drink despite advice to stop and that this was not the first time he had been to the hospital for vomiting blood. She let us know that he had been in the ICU and had to have blood transfusions before. He was hypotensive, tachycardic, radial pulse was weak and thready and his skin was ashy gray.

Within the first 30 seconds of assessment, we knew that he had lost a lot of blood and could go into cardiac arrest in a matter of minutes if we did not figure out how to stop the bleeding and replace some of the blood he had lost. This was critical and every second counted.

Within the first 30 seconds of assessment, we knew that he had lost a lot of blood and could go into cardiac arrest in a matter of minutes if we did not figure out how to stop the bleeding and replace some of the blood he had lost. This was critical and every second counted.

I got a second large bore IV established, drew labs, and double checked that he had IV fluids flowing wide open to keep his tank full until we could get some blood products from the blood bank. It was the type of scenario where we could not afford to wait for the lab to verify his blood type before starting blood transfusions. His condition dictated that we begin transfusion immediately.

The ERP ordered a red box, which is a midsized cooler full of various blood products that we could use to save his life. The danger of using a red box is that none of the blood products are cross matched to the patient's blood type and there is a higher risk of the patient suffering a transfusion reaction. In this case, the risk of him dying outweighed the risk of a reaction.

At this point, the ERP had left the bedside and I was alone with the patient's wife. For the purposes of this story, we will call her Sue. Sue looked exhausted. Her eyelids were puffy from crying. The whites of her eyes were red from stress and lack of sleep. It appeared as though her husband's alcoholism had worn down her spirit. A look of hopelessness had long since drowned the joy from her eyes. The sparkle that once shone from her face had been replaced by a lackluster expression.

I made polite conversation with her while I worked. She had graciously taken on the role of holding a fresh emesis bag for her husband while I prepared the blood tubing, adjusted the monitor for more frequent monitoring, and caught up on charting.

Sue shared with me that she and her husband had been married for over 20 years and she had seen him destroy his health and their relationship with alcohol for the last 15. He listened wearily as she confessed that she was afraid that this would finally be the time that he lost his life to alcohol. Tears quietly flowed down her cheeks as she looked at her husband and back at me. I could tell that she had a lot of love for the man in the hospital gurney. I could also see the sadness in her eyes as she watched him suffer.

My heart ached for Sue. Her husband was in a tremendous amount of pain but there was nothing that I could give him to ease his suffering that would not compromise his already fragile blood pressure. It was a dismal situation that hinged on GI coming to do a scope that would hopefully stop the bleeding.

Normally, an ER tech would support the lifesaving efforts, but since we were so slammed that day, it was just Sue and I in the room with her husband. I was so grateful that she was helping her husband wipe the blood off his face and was standing at the ready with a fresh emesis bag in hand. I had also set up the suction and had it turned on with the yankauer tucked under his pillow where we could reach it easily if needed.

We were in a moment of calm in between storms. She shared with me that he had already had four episodes of vomiting before he reached the hospital and it was nothing but bright red blood.

At that moment, the charge nurse was on her way to the blood bank to pick up our first red box and the ERP was waiting for a return call from the GI doc. The patient's vitals were somewhat stable for the moment and he was resting, his head relaxed back on the gurney.

Sue and I stood in silence, looking at her husband and looking at each other. We felt mutual sadness as we took him in. His ash gray skin sagged from his sunken cheeks. His eyes recessed unnaturally deep in his face. Blood clots clung to the stubble of hair on his chin. A single tear trailed from the corner of his eye.

Alcoholism had overcome this man and I knew in the depths of my being that Sue may be right. This may be the day he lost the war against alcoholism; his life the price to be paid. Sue let out a long, deep sigh and as she looked back at me, I nodded at her. Sue and I had just entered into an unspoken agreement that we were now a team. We stood together, united to support her husband in his very desperate situation.

Just as the charge nurse entered the room, Sue's husband began to moan. Sue looked at me and said, "Here we go again". She knew that I was about to witness another terrible bout of bloody vomiting. I sat the gurney up a little taller, and tossed a towel over his chest while she held the emesis bag closer to his face.

What came next was one of the most forceful exorcisms of bright red blood that I had ever seen. The charge nurse and I looked at each other and we both knew that death was closing in fast. Blood surged from his mouth, hitting the bottom of the vomit bag with such impact that Sue almost lost her grip. An involuntary "Ooh!" escaped my mouth. My eyes widened to match the expression of shock on my face.

Sue stood steadfast as wave after wave of blood exploded from her husband's mouth. I considered speaking words of comfort to them both. I felt compelled to reassure them that the blood products were infusing; that they were sure to help. But my words died in my throat, turned hollow by the cold hard facts as imminent death lingered in the air.

There were no words that could offer comfort. What remained was simply my silent presence. I gently held the patient's wrist to help him keep his arm straight so the blood could enter his vein as quickly as possible.

I observed Sue in admiration. I could not imagine the ravaging effects alcoholism had created in their marriage and, as exhausted as she was, she stayed by his side, hands slippery with his blood as she continued to hold the emesis bag.

When he finally stopped vomiting, there was about 700 cc of blood in the emesis bag. That was more than the unit of blood that was currently being infused into his vein. Sue and I watched the monitor nervously as his heart rate continued to increase and the next reading showed a dangerous dip in blood pressure. We exchanged concerned glances as I put a pressure bag on the blood products in hopes that we could get enough blood into him to replace what had come out in time to keep his system from failing.

I used the second line that the paramedic had placed to hang another bag of blood product. As the monitor cycled every 2.5 minutes, Sue and I anxiously watched the screen, her husband, and each other—silently praying that the reading would be enough to indicate that he would be ok.

He rested back on the gurney again, shoulders slouched in exhaustion, his breath shallow. I opened up another fresh emesis bag as she threw the last one in the trash and used a washcloth to wipe her hands and his chin. Her tears flowed even faster now and my heart ached for her. Blood transfusions continued to flow in two lines.

The last blood pressure reading on the monitor was too low for comfort and his heart rate continued to be tachycardic. I prepped another set of tubing for more blood products and called the ERP to report what I had just witnessed and to inquire about the GI team. The more time that passed without the GI team coming to intervene, the closer this man was to death.

That call brought bad news. The GI team would not come until we could stabilize him more. My heart sank into the pit of my stomach, as I knew that the blood products we were pouring into his veins were just a temporary fix. It was like trying to gas up a car that had a huge hole in the gas tank. The only solution was to repair the hole as continuing to pump gas was simply wasting gas.

The ERP said that the next step was to have him admitted to the ICU. I knew that we could easily be waiting another 45-60 minutes before a bed was available and we could transfer him to the floor. In the meantime, the ERP ordered a second red box of blood products and I called the charge nurse to run to the blood bank again.

Sue sat wearily on the rolling stool that was at the bedside. We were in another moment of calm. The patient looked awful. His skin color had gone from pale ashy gray to almost white. His hands and arms were freezing cold. His eyes were closed and his mouth hung open. His tongue was a dehydrated mass, shriveled in the floor of his mouth. If it weren't for the monitor softly beeping and the slow rise and fall of his chest, I would have thought that he was a corpse.

Sue and I watched as the monitor revealed the newest reading. His blood pressure had started recovering and we shared a collective sigh of relief.

I reached over and offered Sue some tissues and my hand as she sat crying. We held hands in silence while we watched her husband rest, periodically checking the monitor to see what the next blood pressure reading would show. Her pain was thick in the air. We held onto each other as he held on to his life.

The second red box of blood products arrived just as the last few drops of the first round were being infused. I opened up new tubing and started infusing more blood when the patient woke up and started moaning again.

This time, I was more prepared for what was about to come. Sue sighed and stood arms outstretched, hands firmly braced for impact. She had stopped crying and just held the bag as she stared blankly at him. She looked defeated. I felt as defeated as she looked. Bright red blood violently erupted from his mouth and nose.

This was merciless. Blood spewed out of him faster than I could infuse it. At some point, his body would give up. The question was whether that would happen in the ER or after he was transferred to ICU. We were fighting a losing battle.

This was merciless. Blood spewed out of him faster than I could infuse it. At some point, his body would give up. The question was whether that would happen in the ER or after he was transferred to ICU. We were fighting a losing battle.

I continued switching out blood products and fluids and infusing as much as quickly as I could. When the vomiting finally stopped, we measured 800 cc of blood. He had almost filled the entire bag to capacity with the blood that poured out of him.

Sue and I looked at each other and I asked her, "If his heart stops, do you want me to start CPR and try to save his life?"

That felt like a stupid question. We both knew that there was not enough blood left in his body to circulate, even if I did do CPR. Tears flooded her face.

"I don't know." She could barely utter a whisper. She looked over at her husband who weakly shook his head back and forth, "No."

I looked into her eyes, and tears began to flow down my face as her heartbreak permeated my being. I stood there, a silent witness to the violent and bloody ending of a 20-year love story.

She sat back down on the stool and took his hand in hers. She kissed his palm tenderly and then put her cheek to the back of his hand, her tears wetting his skin. He was so weak he couldn't even muster the strength to respond. I stood at the bedside, my cheeks damp with tears. Even though I had done everything in my power, it was not enough to save him.

The ICU nurse knocked on the door frame, alerting us to their arrival. I helped Sue place a few items in a patient belongings bag and handed her the box of tissues and an extra emesis bag to take with her. She set the items on her husband's lap and reached out to give me a hug. We embraced for a few seconds, as tears streamed from our eyes.

She whispered a shaky, "Thank you," in my ear.

I whispered, "You're welcome" in hers. We exchanged one more look and forced smiles as she left to go upstairs with the ICU nurse.

Once he arrived on the floor, the decision was made to place him on comfort care with DNR orders and he passed away about 10 minutes later. Another painful ending of a life and the suffering of a loved one. No matter how much you expect that you will witness death or how prepared you may be, contending for a life that you know will be extinguished, leaves a scar.

I will never forget Sue or her husband. I will never forget going to the bathroom and letting my tears flow for a few minutes. I will never forget the sadness in my heart as I recalled Sue's tears and the tender way Sue had kissed her husband's palm as she accepted the reality that his life was at an end. The hopelessness in my belly as I looked at his ghostly sunken face and felt his cold hand. The frustration that welled up inside of me knowing that everything I did was simply prolonging the inevitability of his death. The anger that roared to life at the suffering created by an addiction unconquered.

I remember standing in that bathroom, looking at myself in the mirror and reminding myself that I had two other patients to check on and a room to clean and prepare for the next emergency. My sadness, hopelessness, frustration, and anger had to be set aside; they had gotten all the time they were going to get.

Suck it up, buttercup! Clean your face, wipe your eyes, and move along.

———

Nursing had become a game of suppression. Suppress the emotional shit storm. Suppress hunger and thirst. Suppress exhaustion.

Suppress the need to go to the bathroom. Stuff it and move on. Someone else was coming to drink from the chronically empty cup.

I have feared losing many patients in my career. Loss is part of the game. I have also feared losing myself.

We are warned of the dangers of contracting a bloodborne illness from infected patients. We are at highest risk for exposure to HIV, Hepatitis B, and Hepatitis C. We are taught how to be cautious and how to protect ourselves from being exposed. We know the risks.

It is not until you are staring at the puncture wound in your finger or you feel the fresh blood splash in your eye that the gravity of the risk really takes hold in your soul.

For me, that moment is as fresh as the memory of yesterday.

An Eye-Full

I took over care at 7:30 am. She was anxious to be discharged. Her fix had long worn off and she was jonesing to get back on the street to find her dealer. It was a sad state, but there was nothing I could do to convince her to stay, to detox, to clean up her life.

I had long since resigned myself to the fact that you can't help people that don't want help.

I sighed and walked into her room, discharge papers in hand. She was dirty and thin from the street life. Her hair was matted into a rat's nest in the back. Her beady eyes darted out of her leathered face, searching for her clothes. Her legs and arms were restless and twitching.

"Good morning. I am Jessica. I am your nurse and I am here to take your IV out so you can be discharged."

She didn't say a word, just held her arm out so I could remove her IV. I noticed the track marks up and down her arm and marveled at the IV that had been placed. The scar tissue from past injections makes it much more difficult to place an IV. I mentally tipped my hat to the nurse that had placed the IV. That was some good work.

I put on gloves and gathered my supplies. Even with my back turned to her, I could feel her anxiety. It buzzed in the air around me. I felt my shoulders tense in reaction to her fidgeting. She sat on the edge of the bed, one leg bouncing urgently.

I sat down on the stool next to her bedside and started the work of removing her IV. As I started peeling up the edges of the tegaderm covering her IV site, she struggled to hold still and became increasingly impatient. I took a deep breath.

"Do your best to hold still for me and I'll be done as fast as possible. I know you are anxious to leave."

With all the tape undone, I was ready to remove the cathlon and cover the IV site with gauze when she said, "Fuck this," yanking her arm away from me. The jerking caused the cathlon to flick back, splashing her blood and saline from the cannula into both of my eyes.

My eyes squeezed shut in an automatic reaction to the foreign liquid. My mind immediately recalled the Hepatitis C diagnosis in her medical history. My heart started racing.

"I may have just contracted Hepatitis C," I thought, my throat imprisoning my breath as I tried to exhale. Panic set in and my mind began to race out of control. In an instant, I imagined myself dying in a hospital bed; yellowed with jaundice and shriveled with regret.

I could see myself dead in a grave, looking up through the lid of the casket, my heart breaking as I watched my children grieve. A loving mother gone too soon.

I opened my eyes, put the gauze over her now bleeding arm, and left the discharge papers on her bed. I was dumbstruck. What was done was done and could not be undone.

This woman was so fixated on her next high that she could not possibly comprehend the gravity of her actions. My stomach churned and I felt nauseated.

I did the only thing that made any sense. I went to the supply closet to gather morgan lenses and saline to flush my eyes. If you don't know what a morgan lens is, picture a big contact with a small hollow tube attached to the middle. That tube connects to a bag of fluid which is used to flush out the eye with copious amounts of liquid. A co-worker helped me place the lenses in my eyes and began flushing.

The room-temperature fluid felt cold on the surface of my eyes, causing my head to whip back into the mattress of the gurney. I exhaled sharply and forced myself to grip the sides of the mattress to keep my hands from ripping out the lenses.

I have tried to wear contacts in the past for vision correction and it was all-out war just to place them in my eyes. One finger would make the approach with the contact while my head backed away, and my other hand swooped in to run interference. My eyes HATED contacts and it was a very dramatic ordeal just to try them out. After many more failed insertion attempts than successes, I decided against contacts and have worn glasses ever since.

Now, there were two massive contacts spewing saline into my eyes like fire hoses. I'm pretty sure I sounded like I was in labor, practicing Lamaze breathing to keep myself steady.

As saline water boarded my eyes, dribbled down the sides of my face, and soaked the back of my head, I did my best to keep my mind on my children. The pain was worth my life. My children deserved to have their momma around as long as possible.

Several months later, I was relieved to be cleared by occupational health when my blood work came back negative for Hepatitis C and any other infectious diseases.

I had survived exposure!

Real Talk

5-minute writing prompt:

Write about a time in your nursing career when you experienced fear.

Reality check

The book 15 Commitments of Conscious Leadership by Jim Dethmer, Diana Chapman and Kelly Klemp, talks about the wisdom of fear. It states that fear is a messenger alerting us of something we should know; whether it is something we refuse to face, or that there is something new to be learned. "Fear invites your full attention and presence."

One of my favorite quotes is, "Fear and faith both demand that you believe in something you cannot see. You choose." Bob Proctor. It reminds me that our minds are powerful. We can choose to stay paralyzed by fear or inspired to move forward in faith. There is always a choice.[4]

Take Action

Join us in the Sh*t They Don't Tell You In Nursing School community and share your stories with us. We offer periodic therapeutic group writing sessions and you are invited!

---

[4] **Source:**
Dethmer, J. Chapman, D. Warner Klemp, K. *The 15 Commitments of Conscious Leadership. 2014.*

Scan QR code to join

https://linktr.ee/jessicasmithdossantos

Shame

Mary C Lamia, PhD wrote an article in *Psychology Today* titled, *Shame: A Concealed, Contagious, and Dangerous Emotion*, in which she defined shame as "a self-conscious emotion [that] informs us of an internal state of inadequacy, unworthiness, dishonor, regret, or disconnection... [and] can lead us to feel as though our whole self is flawed, bad, or subject to exclusion..." [Psychology Today]

I remember feeling this way in my career: Ashamed, unworthy, inadequate, flawed. As I explored what I wanted to share in this section, another poem was born.

The Prison of Shame

Imprisoned in your own mind,
Shame makes the eyes blind.

Inadequate. Unworthy. Isolated. Alone.

Shoulders slouch down, face in a frown,
Stuck in shame, one is likely to drown.

Inadequate. Unworthy. Isolated. Alone.

Feeling less than, worthless, no value to add,
Left drained of energy, lifeless, sad.

Inadequate. Unworthy. Isolated. Alone.

Compared and found lacking in your own mind's eye,
Feeling oppressed, trapped, closed in by the lie.

Inadequate. Unworthy. Isolated. Alone.

The dark whispers of an imbalanced perception
Seek to keep you trapped in the fabrication of deception.

Inadequate. Unworthy. Isolated. Alone.

The weight in the pit of your stomach revealed,
A pain you don't deserve that begs to be healed.

Inadequate. Unworthy. Isolated. Alone.

You are adequate. You are worthy. You are not on your own.
Take my hand, I am here, I see you, you are known.

———————

At one point in my nursing career, I had become a master at numbing my emotions. What looked like a totally composed professional, was really a nurse who purposely refused to feel and who wore a mask that told the world that everything was fine.

I would have described myself as someone who had figured out how to govern the highs and lows. I realize now that I was totally delusional about my mental and emotional state. The truth was, I had figured out how to NOT FEEL. I was numb.

I would have described myself as someone who had figured out how to govern the highs and lows. I realize now that I was totally delusional about my mental and emotional state. The truth was, I had figured out how to NOT FEEL. I was numb.

I wasn't governed or aware. I was checked out. I thought that was a good thing; that not feeling made me bulletproof and more effective as a nurse. Maybe it did when I was at work.

But behind closed doors, I was an emotionally dysfunctional mess. Trapped in my own perception. Believing that I was flawed, bad, wrong, and disgraceful fueled a lie that I deserved to be alone. My eyes were blind and I concluded that I was unworthy of connection. The ultimate suppression and repression of all that I was.

Ray, the Homeless Veteran

My community had a large homeless population and many of them happen to have soul stains deeper and darker than ours from serving in the name of freedom for our country. Veterans have also learned to numb because the pain of feeling the depth of emotions from the things they had done and seen, was too big a burden to bear. For many, numbing meant illegal substance abuse and addiction, which then led to homelessness and social dysfunction. For the purpose of this story, we will call my patient Ray. Ray was brought in from the streets by ambulance.

It was the tail end of winter and the local police had noticed that he had been laying in the same place on the streets for more days than was considered normal. The officer called an ambulance to check on him and the ambulance crew brought him to me.

His vital signs were stable, but he was lethargic and reeked of alcohol, urine, feces, and general filth. He was a man of few words and was compliant, but generally disinterested in anything I did or said. I had no idea when his last meal was or the last time he had cleaned his body. All I knew was that he smelled disgusting and his blue jeans were primarily brown, stained with feces.

He was an alcoholic and had been suffering from abdominal pain and diarrhea for several days. Each beverage came out the other end almost as quickly as it went down. One accident led to a couple of days of shitting and urinating in his own pants. I guess he figured the damage was already done after the first accident, and with no fresh pants or a way to clean himself, it was just easier to lay there and let it happen. Like the poem, he was feeling less-than, worthless; as though he had no value to add.

Feeling inadequate and unworthy left him in my room with pants so stiff with filth that I had to dump warm water on them and let them sit for about 15 minutes before I could even begin to take them off.

I would be lying if I said I was compassionate or empathetic—I was neither.

I was uninterested, detached, and annoyed at the whole situation. I was busy judging him in my mind for being a shitbag and not doing a better job of taking care of himself. For being such a heathen. For not tackling his alcoholism. For being weak. For shitting himself for days on end and apparently not caring.

I was going down a mental list of all the ways his lack of self-care was inconveniencing my day. Comparing, and finding him lacking.

You may be doing a little judging of your own right now. You may be thinking that I was a terrible nurse. You may be thinking that you can't imagine yourself thinking those things about another human, especially one so obviously in need of some TLC. Or you may see yourself in my story.

Maybe you remember a time when you were checked out, uninterested, and judgmental toward your patient. Regardless of where your mind may be wandering right now, I want you to know that you are not always going to be positive, optimistic, or feel like caring for the people you're assigned to.

The places where your mind wanders in these moments are neither good nor bad, but are feedback; a pulse check of your own mental health. A reminder that your thoughts are powerful messengers and deserve attention.

As I removed Ray's pants, it was painfully obvious that the once liquid fecal matter had dried to his skin. The hard-crusted stool wiped away to reveal raw, red, bumpy flesh that resembled a bad diaper rash. Cleaning him was going to be challenging for me and painful for him, no matter how gentle I tried to be.

I soaked him in warm water and tried my best to wipe gently, he protested with each skillful wipe.

"Ouch!"

"Fuck lady, be gentle."

"God damn it!"

"Shit! That hurts!"

My mind continued demeaning him each time he objected, silently calling him names for being such a pain in my ass. I let out a long, loud sigh and muttered a half-hearted apology in response to each protest.

Lost in my mental persecution, I had forgotten why I had become a nurse. I snapped to presence when his filthy hand caught my exposed wrist and I froze as I looked into his eyes.

TRUTH BOMB ───────────────────────────

For the first time since he had arrived,
he held my gaze; I actually SAW him.
Now conscious of the pain and defeat
on his face, the tortures in his being
gripped my consciousness. With
the lens of my criticism removed,
he transformed from a homeless
inconvenience covered in crap, to a man
drowning in shame. My heart ached.

For the first time since he had arrived, he held my gaze; I actually SAW him. Now conscious of the pain and defeat on his face, the tortures in his being gripped my consciousness. With the lens of my criticism removed, he transformed from a homeless inconvenience covered in crap, to a man drowning in shame. My heart ached.

Looking into his soul, I finally appreciated the immense emotional pain he was suffering. My inner critic back peddled. That judgy voice that had been going on and on about how horrible he was, suddenly had nothing to say. For a moment, we connected as humans and I realized how much he was hurting inside. He said to me, "Do you know why I drink so much and shit myself?"

"No," I replied, meekly.

Tears welled up in his eyes and with a thick, wavering voice, he said, "Because I dropped bombs on children and women and old people and got paid by the United States of America to do it. I killed mommas with babies in their arms and grandmas. I flew over and hit a button like it was nothing and then got told I was a hero. I wasn't a hero. I was a fucking murderer. Those women and children were no threat to our freedom. They were innocent and I killed them all. I killed them all."

I stood there, with his chilled fingers clinging to my bare wrist, tears rolling down my cheeks at the agonizing pain in his confession. I was humbled and raw; my ability to feel temporarily awakened. My inner critic felt the sharp slap of guilt for having judged him so harshly. For being so brutally critical. For having been so uninterested in this intoxicated, suffering, rash-covered human being. For feeling inconvenienced by his pain. I had no words. We held eye contact, tears flowing out of our eyes as we looked at each other.

"Do whatever you want. Be rough. I deserve it." he said as he released my wrist.

Now, I was the shitbag. Making up stories in my mind so I didn't have to acknowledge his pain. Judging him to save my own comfort. Numbing my curiosity with head trash so my heart didn't have to know his wound. Not caring about the pain that would drive him to drink himself senseless and be ok with defecating on himself because my ragged and hidden heart couldn't stand to bear witness to his suffering.

When my inner critic stopped judging him, she turned her attention to me.

"You call yourself a nurse?"

"He came to you in one of his worst moments and a time of need and all you did was judge him and let out your disapproval in the form of long loud sighs and half-hearted apologies. Shame on you."

"You didn't even take the time to see him."

"All you saw was an inconvenience. A smear on society."

"You completely dehumanized him."

"You are selfish, broken at the core, and unworthy of the title of Nurse."

This wasn't all that my inner critic had to say, but I think you get the point. Compared and found lacking in my own mind's eye. With those words constantly chattering in my head, I finished my shift as quietly as I possibly could. I tucked tail out the back door as soon as I had given report to the night shift nurse.

I drank wine and ate chocolate in the shower that night and cried like I hadn't cried in a very long time. He had woken up my sad. Some of it received the dignity of being felt. The rest of it was drowned in the high of chocolate and the intoxication of wine.

I faked an illness and called in sick to work the next day, feeling unworthy of caring for another human being.

I questioned my personality, my morals, and my being, and found that I came up too short to be a contribution.

I was so ashamed of myself as I
remembered how it felt to look into his
eyes as he shared his misery. My mind
recycled how horrible I felt for having
judged him, as I sat in the discomfort of
my dysfunctional thoughts. I questioned
my ability to care about others.
My numbness had been ripped open,
exposing my sadness and it was hard.

I was so ashamed of myself as I remembered how it felt to look into his eyes as he shared his misery. My mind recycled how horrible I felt for having judged him, as I sat in the discomfort of my dysfunctional thoughts. I questioned my ability to care about others.

My numbness had been ripped open, exposing my sadness and it was hard.

In retrospect, I realize that Ray was such a gift to me. His shame was a mirror for my shame and it helped me wake up to all the ways that being proud of myself for being "emotionally in check" was a complete lie that I had allowed myself to believe.

Ray helped me see that I was anesthetized, disinterested, apathetic, and indifferent. He helped me realize that numbness had stolen my ability to connect with others and robbed me of my empathy. His vulnerability allowed me to be vulnerable and to connect to my feelings again. He helped me recognize how mortally burned out I was as a human and helped me see that I had let myself go too far.

He woke me up to desiring to do better, to be better for myself and for the people in my life. I will forever be grateful to Ray.[5]

---

[5] **Source:**
Lamela, M. (2011). Shame: A Concealed, Contagious, and Dangerous Emotion (Psychology Today)

Real Talk

5-minute writing prompts:

Write about a time when you were stuck in shame and judging yourself as unworthy, less than, inadequate, dishonorable, flawed, bad, or wrong.

Write about the gifts that shame gave you. What did it wake you up to? How did it support you in your growth?

Reality Check

Shame is part of the rich tapestry of human emotions. Feeling shame is normal; being swallowed by it is dysfunctional and maladaptive. Shame has gifts if you are willing to look for them. Shame gave me back my humanity. It humbled me to my judgment and helped me own my disconnection. Shame grounded me in the present and ripped the Band-Aid off of my lies. It awakened my vulnerability and called me to the carpet of creation. Don't ever doubt that shame can also be a great gift for you if you accept it.

Take Action

If you feel stuck in shame and struggle to see the gifts, schedule a free 20-minute coaching session. I'm here for you!

Scan QR code to schedule

https://linktr.ee/jessicasmithdossantos

Psychoglycemia in the ER

Psychoglycemia: (adjective) mental psychosis caused by low blood sugar. I totally made that up, but if you have been a nurse for any amount of time, you would know it's a real thing. In the spirit of lightening the mood, I want to share with you one of my psychoglycemic moments.

I was nine hours into a 12 hour shift and I had not eaten, drank water, or gone to the bathroom. It was nonstop chaos that day, and I was bordered on hangry. HANGRY! My hands were sticky inside of the gloves I hadn't even had a chance to remove from my last discharge when I heard the overhead page;

"REMSA to 29. ETA 5 minutes. Security has been notified." You know that when security had been called in advance, there was a real rodeo about to go down.

I rushed to the linen closet to grab some fresh sheets and a gown for the room and begged for a cleaning rag from the housekeeper. She was overwhelmed and I knew she wouldn't be able to clean the room in time for the patient who was only 5 minutes out. I furiously scrubbed the gurney when I realized my armpits were soggy. One whiff too close gave away the fact that I had forgotten to put on deodorant.

"Awesome," I thought to myself, shaking my head in disgust. "I am starving, I stink, and all hell is about to break loose."

I had just finished tucking the fresh sheet over the corner of the mattress when I caught sight of the entourage of paramedics, law enforcement officers, and hospital security guards pushing a gurney toward my room. Restrained to the ambulance stretcher by the wrist and ankles was a filthy dirty and nearly naked man, fighting to break free. He spewed a long line of verbal profanities directed at every one and yet no one at the same time. A spit hood was secured around his neck; it covered his face and made him look like an alien. As they rolled closer, I realized that the inside of this man's spit hood was saturated with thick, yellow phlegm.

Ugh, fucking gross.

I cringed at the realization.

I stepped to the side to get report from the paramedic as the team of security and law enforcement wrestled the wild man onto the hospital gurney. He continued his screaming word vomit of profanities at high volume.

The report went something like this: "He is a 56-year-old man who was apparently creating a very loud disturbance in his apartment, which prompted his neighbors to call 911. When we arrived on scene, we observed the patient on the ground in the hallway being restrained by several law enforcement officers, screaming and yelling as you see him here. His apartment was wrecked. Furniture was overturned, clothes, magazines, and trash littered the floor. The place reeked of urine. He has been screaming something about the government spying on him and putting bugs in his apartment to monitor him. We suspect he is high on stimulants. We were unable to obtain a full set of vital signs en route. He is combative. He is strong and has been difficult to control. We have been unable to obtain a medical history. Do you have any questions?"

I exhaled all my disappointment and shook my head side to side. I knew that asking if they could take him to another hospital was out of the question at this point. After the man was safely restrained and the entourage left, I was on my own to get him checked in.

I took a deep breath and walked back into the room with the vitals machine. I proceeded with my usual greeting, "Hello sir, my name is Jessica, you are in the emergency room and I will be your nurse today. I need to take your blood pressure."

I hesitated, surprised because he had stopped screaming. I continued, "I am going to put this blood pressure cuff around your arm and I need you to hold still."

He remained still while I put the cuff around his arm, watching me intently through the snot-saturated net stuck to his face. Then he said, "Look at that pretty little mouth. You should get down on your knees and wrap those lips around my cock."

WHAT?!

I rocked back on my heels, shocked and offended.

THAT. WAS. IT!

I snapped. He was the straw that finally broke this camel's back.

Those two sentences sent me over the edge, my ability to maintain my composure for another second was annihilated. My hands clenched in tight fists and I nearly screamed at him, "Excuse me!? What did you just say? If you are going to talk to me that way, you had best pull my hair and make it worth my while. But since you can't because you are tied up, I suggest you keep your mouth shut."

I realized I had been waving one of my fists in his face as if to say, "Say another word and you will be eating my knuckle sandwich."

The patient's jaw dropped in surprise, as did mine. As soon as my hypoglycemic brain registered what had just come out of my mouth, I was horrified.

—————————————————————————

The psychoglycemia and 9 grueling hours of taking care of patients had officially broken that filter that should have existed between my brain and my mouth to keep those sorts of things from coming out!

The psychoglycemia and 9 grueling hours of taking care of patients had officially broken that filter that should have existed between my brain and my mouth to keep those sorts of things from coming out!

I had all but propositioned and threatened a psychotic restrained patient. Mortified, I turned on my heels and scurried out of the room, closing the door behind me. My eyes landed on the nurse's station and I caught a few of my co-workers looking at me with raised eyebrows. They had obviously heard my interaction.

I looked them all squarely in the faces and said, "I am walking away for a minute. He will be fine until I get back." I went to the breakroom, peed, and chugged the protein shake that I had packed for breakfast.

I took a moment to reflect on the fact that my psychoglycemic nurse personality was akin to a foul-mouthed Amy Schumer character. Good to know. I closed my eyes, shook my head, and sighed. What a mess.

I think we can all safely agree that, even with nearly superhuman emotional composure, there are moments that will all-out break us.

That little unprofessional outburst allowed my frustration to spew out, unsuppressed and uninterrupted. Honestly, it felt GOOD! It gave me a glimpse of what it could look like if I just gave myself permission to feel the feels. Sure, maybe it wasn't the most appropriate place or time, but it was healthy processing. I acknowledged my frustration, gave it a name and a voice, and set it free. No repressing my irritation, no holding on to resentment, no binging on food or alcohol. Just a good old outburst, and I was good to go!

You would think that this would have triggered some spark of awareness in my mind that helped me recognize that I had not been honoring my feelings, but actually suppressing them.

You might think that this would be a teachable moment when I stopped seeing emotional composure and endurance as something to be proud of and started seeing them for what they were: ineffective coping strategies. You might even think that, at that moment, I would have recognized that I didn't need sugar or alcohol to feel better about what had just happened. A little honest venting fixed it. But I didn't connect the dots. I was still subscribing to the persona of nurses being superheroes who didn't show emotions.

Real Talk

5-minute writing prompts:
  Write about a time when you were psychoglycemic.

Reality Check

"When hungry and angry collide, the hangry is real." Mary Beth Albright

Take Action

I can look back now and laugh at that unprofessional moment in my career. We know you have a psychoglycemia story or two up your sleeve! We encourage you to share your stories in our community!

Scan QR code to join

https://linktr.ee/jessicasmithdossantos

Guilt:

Guilt is one of those emotions that can tear you apart from the inside, destroy your self-esteem, and undermine your confidence as a nurse.

In the ER, feelings of guilt are oftentimes associated with events in which the outcomes are finite. The only opportunity is the option to talk about how things might have been done differently. I have spent many nights in the bottom of a bottle, praying that the universe would not be so cruel as to put me in a situation to have to be faced with doing it again because the first time around was just too hard.

Baby Girl

Trigger warning: This content may cause some intense emotions. If you are concerned about being triggered, refer to the PAUSE THE HUSTLE section now and at any time throughout this book.

The rule of thumb when it comes to drownings is as follows: "They are not dead until they are warm and dead".

It is imperative to warm the patient to normal body temperature before ceasing resuscitative efforts and calling the time of death.

When we received the radio report that we were about to receive a 23-month-old female drowning victim with CPR in progress, I was still new to the role of Trauma Nurse. I had passed the Trauma Nursing Core Course (TNCC) certification exam. I was an Emergency Nurse Pediatric Course Instructor (ENPC-I). I had even earned the title of Board-Certified Emergency Nurse (BCEN). I had enough letters behind my name and enough training on the clock to work unsupervised as a Trauma Nurse.

This was both my first drowning victim and my first pediatric trauma. I prepped the trauma bay, turning on the warming lights as I mentally prepared for what I was about to do. My heart raced, and my palms were sweaty. I hadn't had enough experience to develop my intuition in a trauma scenario and I was nervous.

Per the report, Baby Girl was left unattended at the water's edge of a lake. When her father came back to check on her, she was fully submerged under the water and unconscious. In a complete panic, he pulled her out of the water, put her in the car, and drove to the nearest hospital he could think of.

I can only imagine the terror in his soul as he drove wildly for help. His lifeless, unconscious daughter in the back seat. Unfortunately, the nearest "hospital" was a rehab center. They were not prepared or equipped to care for an unresponsive, pulseless child. The staff activated emergency services and started CPR in the lobby while waiting for the medic crew to arrive.

We estimated that she had been pulseless for 8-10 minutes before CPR was started and it was at least 15-20 minutes total between the time she was found submerged to the time the ambulance crew took over care.

We were unable to determine how long she had been unconscious and submerged in the water.

The outcome was grim at best from the very beginning. She had already gone too long without a pulse before she even reached the trauma bay.

We transitioned her from the EMS gurney onto the trauma bay table. Warm blankets under her body; warming lights on above. We continued CPR, verified intubation, and gave the emergency medications at the appropriate intervals. We worked her for what seemed like an eternity, my fingers flying over the keyboard, documenting every intervention. The one thing I had not documented was a normal temperature.

"She is not dead until she is warm and dead," the mantra raced through my mind. I glanced over at my seasoned co-worker with the question flashing in my eyes, "Shouldn't we get her warmer?"

She glanced back at me, her brows raised in affirmation. She reached over and patted my arm as if to say, "Trust the process. We got this."

I nodded an unspoken agreement as I shifted my gaze back to the trauma team. Their expert hands moved in a revival dance; pulsing, compressing, expertly willing Baby Girl back to life.

The tears that had been dammed up behind my swollen eyelids flowed forth as the physician waved his hand in a sign to stop. The team stood breathless and silent around her small limp body.

"She isn't dead until she is warm and dead," repeated the voice in my mind.

I had never documented a normal temperature on her. They were all below normal.

Despite the knot in my guts and the question in my head, I remained quiet. Something about being new to the trauma team and not feeling comfortable to speak up kept me mute. That, and the fact that she had already gone so long without a pulse before she even made it to us, meant that she had likely already sustained a massive anoxic brain injury.

"Time of death, 17:02," the Doctor announced. We stood together in a collective moment of silence in honor of Baby Girl's life. With heavy hearts, we cleaned up the trauma bay in preparation for her parents.

"She isn't dead until she is warm and dead," the voice in my mind spoke again.

I went to the blanket warmer and removed two blankets, preparing to swaddle her. I wanted her to look peaceful when the social worker brought her family to the bedside. My hands trembled as I carefully lifted her body off the cold metal trauma table and pressed her against my chest, a sob escaping my throat as I wrapped the warm blanket around her back. I held her close as my tears fell onto her downy brown hair.

I gently laid her petite body back on the table. My tears flowed faster as I admired her features, much like my daughter's when she was three.

Soft, dark eyelashes, plump cheeks. A dainty button nose. Delicate lips. I felt my heart break as my mind drifted.

What if this was my daughter?

Another sob escaped as the tech rubbed my back, "Shhh," she said. "Wipe your tears. The family will be in soon."

I worked to compose myself for what was yet to come; wondering if I was strong enough to hold space for her parent's pain as they said goodbye.

The social worker escorted the parents into the trauma bay. The father's wails were a sound I will never ever forget. It was a tortured scream that only a father who was witnessing the corpse of his 23-month-old daughter could make. The burden of her death howled from his throat.

Hot tears rolled down my face witnessing his pain. My eyes went from Baby Girl—lifeless on the trauma table—to Mom who stood silent, pale, and stoic, to Dad. His hands gripped the side of the trauma table so hard that his knuckles were white. His tortured screams echoed through the halls of the ER. I watched his soul break into a million pieces, and it felt as if mine was breaking too.

I was in a rough transition of life. I had just separated from my husband with whom I shared custody of our 5-year-old daughter and our 6-year-old son. My babies were with their dad for the weekend. Standing in that trauma bay, witnessing that father's soul break into a million pieces, I could not stop the tears from streaming down my face. I could not separate his pain from the imagination of how I would feel if that were my baby girl's limp body lying on that table. I wanted to run out of that trauma bay and hold my babies tight.

My warm, alive, healthy, breathing babies.

There were no words that would comfort this family in their agony. There was nothing for us to do except silently witness their last moments with their deceased daughter, hear their tortured sobs, and do our best to remain professional.

The air was thick with emotion. Our hearts broke for the family and we carried deep sadness as a team at the loss of her life. We knew the odds were not in our favor from the very beginning, but when the life of a child is on the line, there is an extra sense of urgency and responsibility for all of us.

"Oh, my God," her mother screamed, "She is breathing!"

We all took a step closer to Baby Girl—wide eyes glued to her chest.

"SHE ISN'T DEAD UNTIL SHE IS WARM AND DEAD!" The mantra screamed in my mind.

"That's a breath," the Doctor announced as we watched her tiny chest rise and fall softly again. "Resume CPR and take her to the Peds Code room! Prepare a catheter for warm bladder irrigation and aggressive warming measures."

I stood there in a daze, watching the team work.

Why didn't I say something sooner?

Why didn't I feel confident enough to use my voice and trust my training?

Why?

My mind punished me for not having spoken up in the trauma bay when we called the time of death the first time around.

I felt an overwhelming sense of guilt and responsibility for never having said a word when the one repeating thought that kept running through my head was, "She is not dead until she is warm and dead."

To our amazement, her heart started spontaneously beating again. Our efforts had worked!

As I watched her parents hugging each other at the bedside—eyes red from crying, hopefully watching the heartbeat on the monitor and looking at their unconscious, but alive baby girl—I cried again; not tears of hope or tears of relief, but tears of horrible, awful guilt.

I had a horrendous knot in the pit of my stomach because I knew that Baby Girl would never ever wake up. Her heart was beating, but she had already suffered too much injury to her brain, and she would never regain consciousness.

I felt like I was being ripped apart from the inside out.

I should have said something.

I should have opened my damn mouth and asked about bringing her temperature back to normal before calling the time of death.

I should have been an advocate for my training and just spoke up.

But I didn't. And here I was, watching her parents hug each other and start to hope for their Baby Girl when I knew she would never, ever recover.

Guilt. Overwhelming, consuming, tearing me apart from the inside, destroying my self-esteem, undermining my confidence.

I felt thoroughly unworthy of all those letters behind my name and that badge attached to my scrubs. I was devastated.

Wine and chocolate wouldn't cut it that night. Truth be told, I never was much of a drinker. I didn't like the feeling of being out of control when I was drunk and I really didn't like the way I felt the next day.

I almost never bought alcohol for myself. I didn't really understand the appeal until I learned that it worked pretty well to shut that shitty hurt feeling off.

The hurt I felt in my heart was immense that day. I stopped by my soon to be ex-husband's house after work to hug my children. While we were having our fair share of differences, he was a decent man and could understand my need to be with the babies that night. I cried the whole drive home, where I was greeted by an empty house. A silent reminder of a family that once was. It was fucking depressing. I stood in the kitchen, tears continued to roll down my face as I glanced up at the liquor cabinet.

I opened the door and bypassed the wine. This pain required something stronger. My hand landed on a bottle of Basil Hayden bourbon.

I was searching for a glass when my eyes landed on a colorful stack of Tupperware cups that I had for my kids. I began to sob again. Somewhere, there was a cabinet with a colorful Tupperware cup that a beautiful Baby Girl had once drank out of; innocently waiting to be discovered to remind a grieving father of his mistake. To remind a mother of her loss. I closed the cabinet, deciding against a cup.

I opened the bottle and took it with me in the shower. It burned good. My nostrils flared, my chest scorched, and I sputtered a little cough after my first swallow. It was strong and I was hopeful.

I leaned back against the shower wall, letting the hot water wash away the tears and the guilt. Burning swig after burning swig, I tried to shut the pain down. I was grateful the bourbon was strong and that I was such a lightweight.

I wept until there was nothing left. I cried and the bourbon numbed. I couldn't drink enough to silence that father's wails in my memory. No amount of bourbon could stop my brain from imagining my own daughter, face down, floating in a lake.

I was sitting on the floor of the shower; the water turned cold. My arms and legs were heavy. My face felt bloated. My eyes were blurry from bourbon and tears.

Somehow, I managed to pull my drenched naked body out of the shower and crawl to bed. I didn't care that I was still wet or that I hadn't brushed my teeth. All I knew was that I was grateful to be numb.

That was my first experience with drinking until I passed out. I woke up several hours later, shivering on top of my bed, head spinning, stomach preparing to hurl. Thankfully, I made it to the toilet before puking my guts up. It burned coming back up just as much as it had burned going down. Except this time, it came back up so forcefully it burned my nostrils, too.

I rinsed my wretched mouth with mouthwash and dragged my sorry naked ass back to bed, dreading the morning.

———

As medical professionals, we sometimes have seconds to make a life-altering decision. One mistake can be one mistake too many. I could have allowed that overwhelming guilt to continue to tear me apart from the inside, destroy my self-esteem, and undermine my confidence, but I didn't.

Like the tattoo on my wrist says, "Can't change it."

I could not change what happened; the only choice I had was to decide how I would learn from it.

From that day forward, no question went unasked, no thought unexpressed. The guilt I felt inside became the gift that took me to a new level of confidence both in my career and in my life.

That Baby Girl, her petite features still etched in my mind even today, reminds me how important it is to trust myself and use my voice. Her death gave me the courage to share this story, to share my grief and the guilt of that moment. She gave me the conviction to speak up no matter what the situation. Her outcome didn't change, but mine did, and for that, I will forever be grateful.

Real Talk

5-minute writing prompt:

Think back to a time when you felt guilty about something that happened in your career. What gift did the guilt give you?

Reality Check

In the same way that a one-sided piece of bread is an impossibility, so is guilt without a gift. The only thing that keeps you from seeing the gift in the guilt is your perception. Let Baby Girl's story be your reminder to speak up.

Take Action

Carrying the burden of guilt without understanding the gift can be torture. You do not have to suffer in silence. I would love to offer you a free 20-minute coaching session. Simply schedule a call.

Scan QR code to schedule

https://linktr.ee/jessicasmithdossantos

Purple Man Junk

None of us are excited about the gross parts of nursing, but we are not naive to what we are getting into either. Human illness is disgusting! Wiping butts, touching other people's private parts, sticking tubes in urethras, noses, and anuses. Listening to stories of how things became stuck in holes where they do not belong (like an apple up the butt that had to be surgically removed—true story). Blood, vomit, sputum, urine, feces, oozing infections, leaking body parts. All expected.

But what about when we encounter something unexpectedly disgusting that nursing school could never possibly prepare us for? I call it a soul stain. Like a skid mark left in a new pair of underwear. When something so gross and unexpected happens, it leaves a stain on the soul.

We have a dedicated area in the ER where all of our acutely ill psychiatric patients are cared for. Those rooms are generally stripped of all equipment, cords, cables, and supplies as a method of keeping our patients and ourselves safe. Most psychiatric patients are mentally unstable and at high risk of harming themselves or others.

Admittedly, it was my least favorite place to work. I felt like a master negotiator all day long. Trying to compromise with people who are not in their right mind is like trying to help a toddler understand the physics of a rocket ship. It generally left me mentally and emotionally exhausted after a 12-hour day.

The ironic part of this whole story is the fact that I wasn't even assigned to this area the day it all went down. Nope! I was actually just innocently passing through on my way to a much-needed and rarely-received lunch break.

Did you catch that!? I was on my way to one of those elusive things called a LUNCH BREAK when a peculiar noise coming from the room on my left caused me to glance over as I walked by.

What I saw made me stop in my tracks. A middle-aged man with his penis and testicles on full display. That in itself wasn't enough to make me stop. It was the fact that his man junk was the color of a deep purple grape.

What I saw made me stop in my tracks. A middle-aged man with his penis and testicles on full display. That in itself wasn't enough to make me stop. It was the fact that his man junk was the color of a deep purple grape. My brain experienced a momentary glitch in which my eyes were involuntarily glued to his Full Monty privates while I tried to figure out why a light tan man had dark purple junk.

When I finally put the pieces together, I groaned in disbelief. He had ripped the hem off of his hospital gown and tied it multiple times, as tightly as he could, around the base of his penis and testicles so that it cut off the circulation. Deep purple man junk explained.

I glanced back at the nurse's station and realized, with a sinking feeling in my stomach, that there was no staff to report to so I could go on about my lunch break. The two nurses who worked in the area were both in other rooms with security trying to contain acutely violent patients.

Looking back on this memory, I judge myself a little bit for having the thought that came next. I hesitated in the hallway wondering to myself, "If I just go in and cover him with a blanket, I wonder how long I have to leave him like that to cause sterility so that he cannot reproduce?"

Savage, I know. My mind wandered to some pretty deep and dark corners in that burned-out season of my career.

I let out a deep sigh, and my shoulders sagged in resignation. There goes the lunch break I was so excited about. I had to save a man from himself.

I grabbed some gloves—instead of that much-anticipated food—and asked one of the security guards to come into the room with me. I knew absolutely nothing about this man other than the fact that he was strangling his manhood and doing a dang good job at it.

I introduced myself, "Hello, sir. My name is Jessica. I am a nurse. I couldn't help but notice you seem to be in a lot of pain and it looks like your penis is in trouble. I am here to help."

The man said, "No! Don't remove it! If any of my life force leaks out, I will DIE!!!"

"His life force?" I contemplated, looking at the security guard for answers as if he possessed some exclusive insight into the enigmatic realm of male physiology that I, as a woman, was unaware of. However, his shrug of confusion indicated that he, too, was baffled.

"Your life force?" I asked the patient.

"YES," he wailed. "My yellow liquid life force! It cannot come out! I can't die this way!"

"Are you talking about your urine?" I tried to understand.

"YES! NO! My life force," he continued to moan in obvious discomfort.

What I think I understood was that he had to urinate and he believed that his pee was his life force. In his mind, if he let any of the urine out, he would indeed die. So, he did the only thing that made sense: ripped the hem off of his gown and tied it around himself as a way of putting a kink in the hose to save his own life.

When I took a moment to reflect on the fact that this thought was so strongly his reality that he was willing to harm his own privates, I realized how difficult life must have been to navigate. To him, this was a matter of life and death and he chose life in the only way that made any sense to him. I simultaneously felt sad for him and so grateful that my mind, while sometimes dark in thoughts, was still in touch with reality.

I went out of the room to grab a urinal and assured him that we would be saving all of his life force in the container and that as long as it was near him, he would live. It took some time to convince him that I was trained in the ways of the life force and that I had experience in such things. I reassured him that he would be ok.

His face sweated as his hands white-knuckled the sheets when he finally agreed to cooperate with letting us remove the cloth tourniquet he had so effectively tied around himself.

I took a deep breath as my gloved hands went in for the rescue. He had wrapped it and tied it in a knot and then wrapped it again and tied another knot. There were at least 10 very tight knots to undo. To my exasperation, he had tied the hem so tightly around himself that I had to use my hemostats to get the knots to loosen.

While I worked, his urine leaked out all over my hands and wrists. Squirting up my arm, past the cuff of my glove and onto my bare skin, then dribbling back down my wrists into my gloves, leaving my fingertips warm and squishy. Fifteen very disgustingly intimate minutes later, Willy was free, and I had a fresh soul stain skid marked on my spirit.

Real Talk

5-minute writing prompt:
    Write about a time when you were unexpectedly disgusted.

Reality Check

"Disgust and resolve are the two great emotions that lead to change." Jim Rohn.

Take Action

Join us in the S**t They Don't Tell You In Nursing School community and share your disgusting story with us!

Scan QR code to join

https://linktr.ee/jessicasmithdossantos

Anger

Anger is the final resting place of your old story and the rich soil for the beginning of the next chapter of your life. The emotional pain of anger that blazes inside of you like wildfire forces you to wake up to what is real. Reality confronts you into making a change; to set a boundary, to have an important conversation, or to settle into a decision.

My final resting place

I remember that day with such clarity. The final resting place for my old story. What had started as a spark several years prior had finally reached a fiery rage. I woke up just before the sound of my alarm and everything in me said "NO!"

Every part of me was wild with anger. It could no longer be contained with chocolate or alcohol. The gale force winds of my life blew the firestorm past the containment of my coping skills as it roared out of control in my being, swallowing me whole, setting every part of me aflame.

Resentment felt like gasoline in my veins, burning its way through, adding fuel to the fire as it gained momentum inside of me, "AAAAAAAHHHHHHHHHHHHHHH!"

I screamed at the ceiling. Tears flowed out of my eyes as my ravenous hands ripped and tore at my bedsheets. My heart pounded in my ears, the veins in my neck bulged under the pressure of my straining muscles. My mind raced as I recalled all the hurt, the guilt, the fear, and the shame in a rapid-fire sequence in my mind.

I had spent so much of my life giving to a career that had taken everything: my time with my children, my joy, my energy, my hustle, my grind, my health, my happiness, my financial stability, my empathy, and even my marriage. The sacrifice was too great and the return insufficient. To the profession, I was just one in a pool of millions. I didn't matter.

"I AM FUCKING DONE!" I roared into the silence of my bedroom. "NO MORE!"

I lay there in my bed, my body flushed red, the sheets sticking to the sweat that had collected on my spine. I felt like a foreigner in my own skin.

"Who am I right now?" I thought to myself.

Deep down in the core of my being, I knew I was burned-out. I showed up to work apathetic and precarious. I knew I could no longer serve a profession that required me to be so completely consumed, with nothing left to give. I knew that if I kept caring for people in this state, I would make a fatal error and endanger the life that had been entrusted to me.

I realized that I was practicing nursing in a dangerous manner; I had become apathetic and precarious. With no skills to navigate the depth of my emotional suffering, using sugar and alcohol as temporary solutions, my thoughts became nasty, my heart turned cold, and I had no fucks left to give—to anyone.

I realized that I was practicing nursing in a dangerous manner; I had become apathetic and precarious. With no skills to navigate the depth of my emotional suffering, using sugar and alcohol as temporary solutions, my thoughts became nasty, my heart turned cold, and I had no fucks left to give—to anyone.

I rolled out of bed, my skin tingling from head to toe as the scorched heat radiated from my body. I inhaled a long, deep breath, catching my air in the aftermath. I squared my shoulders. I knew what I needed to do. I was putting in my two-week notice. I was done.

I had a clear "NO". I had known for a long time that my life was out of alignment with who I was and what I was put here to do. I knew that the profession of nursing was no longer in service of my purpose. I knew that this ending was the necessary beginning of the next chapter of my life.

———————

I was no longer willing to stay stuck. I was no longer willing to give without return. I was no longer willing to invest my time, energy, and my health. I was ready to take ownership of my experience. Today was the finale of my ER career and the beginning of the wide-open spaces that were the blank pages of my future, ready to be written. I felt free.

"Our personal and professional lives can only improve to the degree that we can see endings as a necessary and strategic step to something better. If we cannot see endings in a positive light and execute them well, the 'better' will never come." Dr. Henry Cloud

Real Talk

5-minute writing prompt:

What is your anger trying to tell you? What is out of alignment, no longer in service, or needs to be changed?

Reality Check

Please don't get me wrong here. I am not encouraging or advocating for you to retire from the profession as I did. I transitioned out of patient care and into a nursing role that parked me behind a desk. I worked an exit strategy, with the assistance of a mentor, for a year before I fully retired. My story may parallel yours in many ways, but the path to your next chapter will be unique to you. What I am advocating for is that you to listen to that raging anger burning inside of you. Lean into the wisdom that is there for you.

"Nature understands [that eradication is occasionally necessary] and is not afraid to destroy something that is no longer sustainable. Destruction opens the possibility for new birth—when a wildfire burns a dead forest, the heat releases the seeds into the newly created fertile soil." Jim Dethmer, et, al.

I encourage you to identify all that is dead inside of you and have the courage to let it burn to the ground so that the seeds of your next chapter can take root in the fertile soil that will be left for your future.

Take Action

Whether you want to feel good about serving people in a holistic way and would like to explore coaching as an avenue to support you in feeling alive, fulfilled, and aligned again; or if you want to do what I did and exit nursing all together, I encourage you to schedule a call with me to explore if coaching could be the next best step for you. I mentor both new and seasoned coaches in the skills required to launch and scale impactful coaching practices.

Scan QR code to schedule

https://linktr.ee/jessicasmithdossantos

WHAT'S YOUR DRUG OF CHOICE?

W hat's your drug of choice? You know what I mean. That thing that you do to try to make yourself feel better when life feels shitty and the emotions are just too hard. That thing that you know isn't necessarily healthy for you, but you do it anyway because it feels better than the hell you are going through.

You might think my drug of choice was alcohol, but you would be wrong. Alcohol was more like a desperate bootie call. It looked good and I had high expectations, but in the end, it was just a letdown and I felt gross afterward.

That was what alcohol was for me. It was an act of desperation with the expectation that I would stop feeling.

My drug of choice was sugar. Specifically, anything chocolate. I learned at a very young age that chocolate never said no and always made me feel good when I needed it the most. It was easy to get my hands on and the rush was almost instantaneous.

The Addiction Begins

My 9-year-old heart broke as I sat on the back porch steps, tears soaking the palms of my hands. My heart was broken. Something was missing. I was not complete.

My faithful border collie, Bud, sat by my side and he looked concerned. He kept whimpering and licking the tears off of my cheeks. I wrapped my arms around him and gave him a big hug, burying my face into his furry chest and sobbing as the questions rattled through my mind, like a rapid-fire gunshot being expelled from an automatic weapon.

Why did he leave me here?
Why couldn't I go with him?
Wasn't I his best friend?
His whole world?
Will he come back to take me, too?

I didn't want to be here without him.

A few days earlier my dad had moved out. My parents were getting a divorce and Dad left. I remembered all the times we spent together, working on cars. He owned an automotive shop and I was always so excited to go to work and help him. I closed my wet eyes and remembered how I would get under the cars with him on the creeper. I liked the wooden one with the red headrest. He would use the black one with the blue headrest.

I cried.

Our shoulders would be touching. I remembered how I loved watching him work. He would patiently explain what he was doing and periodically look over at me and smile. I was part of his world and he was part of mine. It was special. I felt special.

I cried harder.

I remembered the way he smelled, the grease and dirt and Dad smell. I loved that smell. It smelled like safety and love and happiness. It smelled like home.

My chest tightened as I gripped the front of my shirt in my fists, grimacing with pain. Something was wrong. Something was missing and it hurt so bad. My throat was thick and I could barely breathe.

I remembered how I felt when I followed Dad's instructions and he praised me for doing a good job. He was so proud of me. I was good. Except now, I was alone because he left.

I cried even harder.

He was gone. And I was here. I felt empty, incomplete, exposed, and insecure.

The sun had started going down and I shivered as the temperature in the air dropped several degrees. I stood up and went into the house, closing the door behind me. I continued to cry. My feet felt heavy, my body drained of strength.

My shoulders slouched and my chest ached. I hated this feeling. Defeated. Empty. Hurting. My breath was shallow and my chest was constricted. This feeling was awful. It was painful to take a deep breath. The thoughts continued.

Why did it hurt so bad?

Why didn't I get to go with him too?

Why did he leave me?

Did he still love me?

I felt ugly. Unworthy. Not enough.

My eyes scanned the kitchen and rested on a pack of Costco muffins. The three-flavor pack with the poppyseed, blueberry, and chocolate flavors. I walked over to the counter and removed a muffin.

I wiped my eyes and my nose with the sleeve of my dirty sweatshirt and looked around for my mom. She was up at the barn with the horses and I knew she would be down soon to start dinner.

No way she would let me eat one of these before dinner.

But she wasn't there. Neither was Dad. My chest tightened again; my breath felt stuck, my face was numb. More tears spilled out of my eyes and down my cheeks. I looked down at the muffin, my vision blurry.

The bottom barely fit in my hand because it was so big. Mom usually cut it into fourths for everyone to share. The sweet chocolate smell made my mouth water with anticipation.

I glanced at the front door and then took a bite of the muffin. I felt my shoulders relax. I closed my eyes as I rolled the muffin over my tongue, feeling the thick chocolate chunks start to melt. I took a slow, deep breath in through my snotty nostrils as the tight feeling in my chest started to release. I inhaled all the way down to the bottom of my lungs.

Again, I felt that familiar feeling like I was back under the car with Dad. I felt better. I let out a sigh of relief.

I sniffed the snot back into my nose and started chewing. Savoring the flavor. The cake was moist, the chocolate sweet. I swished the thick liquid confection around in my mouth, letting it coat my teeth and the inside of my cheeks. I swallowed and took a big, long, deep, satisfying breath of air as the pain in my chest subsided.

My face flushed warm as my body continued to relax. I walked over to the kitchen table and sat down, muffin in hand. I glanced at the front door, wondering if Mom would come in and catch me. I knew I would be in trouble if she saw what I was doing.

I looked back at the muffin and I wanted more. More of that feeling. I wanted to feel safe again. Happy. Special. Like I did when I was with Dad. I took another huge bite, but this time I didn't savor it like the first one. I chewed quickly, feeling the waves of feel-good wash over me. Dopamine dumping in my brain.

It wasn't exactly the same as when I was with Dad, but it was close. Kinda. It was definitely a lot better than feeling the pain of abandonment. I had temporarily forgotten that Dad was gone. I kept glancing at the front door, knowing Mom would be coming in any minute and I didn't want this feeling to stop.

I ate greedily until the whole thing was gone. I stared down at the empty muffin paper, swallowing the last bite. My tongue slid over the sugary film on my teeth, scouring for the last taste of chocolaty goodness. I felt full and content.

I scraped the crumbs off the table into the muffin paper and put them in the trash can, thoughtfully hidden under a piece of old tin foil in hopes that Mom wouldn't realize what I had done. I glanced over at the counter and counted two chocolate muffins left.

Maybe Mom wouldn't notice that there was one missing. I felt a little shameful and guilty about what I had done, but, at the same time, I wanted to eat a second one. I liked the way it made me feel and I was starting to miss Dad again. My heart felt heavy.

The addiction had begun. The love-hate relationship with sugar was birthed in one moment of pain dulled by chocolate.

———

In healthcare, chocolate was everywhere. All the time. In the candy jar at the charge desk, in the supervisor's office, on the counter in the breakroom, in the vending machine, at the coffee shop, and by the register in the cafeteria. Everywhere.

It never told me no and always made me feel good when I needed it the most. It was easy to get my hands on and the rush was almost instantaneous. It made the lows more tolerable and the highs gloriously higher.

Real Talk

5-minute writing prompt:
   What's your drug of choice?

Reality Check

I have lost friends in the medical field to drug overdoses and complications of alcoholism. I have watched them suffer from diabetes, heart disease, and obesity because of food addiction. I myself have contended with food, alcohol, promiscuity, and retail therapy as the drugs that kept me numb and high. We see each other abusing, we watch each other struggle, and yet we feel justified in our mechanisms because of the shit we do every day. Not because we think it is ok, but because we don't know another way. If you are currently struggling with an addiction or a destructive habit, please know that you are not alone. I know your pain and I am here for you. There is a better way.

Take Action

While I am not trained in substance abuse and I do not do recovery counseling, I am here for you as a safe, nonjudgmental place to be open and honest about your challenges. I believe there is a healthier, happier life for you. Take advantage of the free 20-minute coaching session.

Scan QR code to schedule

https://linktr.ee/jessicasmithdossantos

PAUSE THE HUSTLE

In nursing school, they omitted the crucial lesson that what we did for ourselves took precedence over everything else we would do for others. What you do for your health, your well-being, and your relationships matters. Your quality-of-life matters. I am here to tell you now, YOU MATTER.

I have pointed fingers at nursing school for not preparing us for the emotional toll this career can have. I have shared some compelling statistic about nursing being a "fertile soil for risk of suicide". I have called out the dangers of misunderstanding the trait of altruism as an identity, and I have given warning about confusing the skillsets of emotional composure and endurance with emotional suppression and numbing.

I made a bold statement in the beginning that this book is meant to empower, prepare, and support you, my fellow Nurse, to first and foremost be your own greatest caregiver.

Now, I have an essential question for you: Are you ready to learn how to release all of that fear, shame, guilt, and anger so that you may feel alive, fulfilled, and fully aligned? If you are, then keep reading.

I realized this for myself: not only had I become a master at numbing my emotions, but I had also developed a strategy of being busy to avoid the hard parts of my life. As long as I was too busy distracting myself with tasks and hustling to get things done, I would not have time to sit in the discomfort of being with my emotions. I was aware of what I was doing, but I didn't know how to break free.

It took hiring a coach to help me see my blind spots, and to identify those stop points. Those moments required me to PAUSE THE HUSTLE so I could leverage the opportunity to do the hard thing: be with my emotions and feel them all the way through to completion.

PAUSE THE HUSTLE is an acronym for the process that has helped me release my feelings so that I may heal. It is also the process that I guide my clients through as they learn to feel their feelings. This process will set you free if you choose to practice it.

- **PAUSE**: Pause, quiet the busy in your mind, and check in with yourself.
- **APPRECIATE**: Appreciate this moment and know that it is OK to be where you are and to feel what you feel. Resist the urge to judge.
- **UNDERSTAND**: Understand that you are safe to feel your feelings.
- **SENSE:** What are you feeling in your body right now? Put your hands on the sensation to locate where your feeling is being held.
- **EMOTION:** What emotion are you feeling right now?
- **TAKE ACTION:** The next step in feeling emotions is to allow the emotions to physically move through the body. If that emotion could move, what movement would it

make? Like a toddler having a tantrum to release anger, or a football player doing a victory dance to release joy, each feeling has a movement. Go ahead; move, dance, contract, wiggle, kick, punch, rock, flail about.

- **HARMONIZE:** Allow your feeling to be heard. Allow it to flow through your vocal cords and to harmonize with the sensations and movements that are coming up for you. The toddler screams to release, the football player lets out a victory whoop, and the teenage girl squeals when she is excited. If your emotion could make a sound, what sound would it make? Let it out! All those weird noises, let them out!

- **EXPRESS:** Commit to releasing the emotion completely by expressing it through movement and sound until the sensation is fully resolved in your body. When you think you are done ask yourself, "Is there any more?"

- **HUMAN:** Congratulations! You are human! Celebrate how normal you are for having emotions and for being willing to express yourself in the ways humans do. Be proud of yourself for putting down the superhero cape to just BE HUMAN! UNPLUG from the seriousness of it all!

- **UNPLUG:** Unplug from the hustle of life.

- **SMILE:** You just did the hardest thing of all. You chose to pause the hustle and prioritize yourself. Be so proud of you—smile!

- **TRUST YOURSELF:** You have always been and always will be your own best guide on this journey. All that is required is trust.

- **LIBERATED**: Learning to release feelings is your liberator.

- **EMPOWERED:** You have everything inside of you that
  you have ever needed. Empowered with the knowledge
  and the skills to feel and release your feelings, you are a
  soul untethered.

Courage to Pause

When I first learned to release emotions rather than suppress
them, it took conscious effort to choose to PAUSE, and practice
a new way of being with myself. Here is what it looked like when
I started learning to PAUSE THE HUSTLE and process sadness.

PAUSE

Pause, quiet the busy in your mind, and check in with yourself.

My mind was racing in a hundred different directions, cycling
through the never-ending to-do lists of my life. I felt like a
hamster stuck in the wheel, my legs running faster and faster,
trying to keep up. Panicking, knowing at any second the wheel
would go too fast and I would lose the race. It would spin me out
of control and leave me panting in the sawdust floor of the cage
that had become my existence. My coach's voice floated through
the blur, "The overwhelmed mind does nothing."

I paused, taking in a long deep breath and held it, willing
the to-do lists to sit down and wait their turn. I exhaled slowly,
commanding my busy mind like a skilled kindergarten teacher.

"Sit down, crisscross applesauce on the carpet, and catch a
bubble."

I inhaled again as the chatter in my mind slowed. I focused my
awareness on the feeling of the air moving through my nostrils

and into my lungs. My heart rate slowed. I let the air out to a count of four. One. Two. Three. Four. "No one is dying right now," I reminded myself. "I am ok."

Overwhelmed, over-committed, and over-scheduled had become my strategy to avoid checking in with my feelings. It was more comfortable to be caught in the anxiety of the hamster wheel than it was to sit with myself. But then I remembered, I MATTER. Not the to-do lists, the commitments, the schedules. ME. It was time for ME to be ok.

APPRECIATE

Appreciate this moment and know that it is OK to be where you are and to feel what you feel. Resist the urge to judge.

As I stood there in the kitchen, breathing, looking at the laundry list of to-dos written on my notepad, my inner critic took advantage of the quiet, "You are better than this. You are capable of so much more. Why can't you just get your shit together and take care of business?"

I sucked in a sharp breath as I felt the tears well up in my eyes. I quickly brushed them away. "Not today," I said out loud. I felt the kindergartners in my mind becoming restless again. Then it struck me.

This is more than one human can get done in a month, much less in one day off between shifts. No wonder I am feeling overwhelmed.

I let my breath out in a woosh and I heard my coach again, "The overwhelmed mind does nothing." I closed my eyes and took in a long, deep breath, held it, and let it out slowly. "I am ok," I said out loud. "I am ok." I nodded in affirmation. It was time for me to be ok.

UNDERSTAND

Understand that you are safe to feel your feelings.

Again, I heard my coach's voice in my mind, "Being busy won't fix it. If it did, you would be ok right now. What do you really need?"

A lump in my throat welled up, choking off my breath. The tears stung hot behind my eyes and overflowed down my cheeks. I needed to be sad. I needed to grieve. I needed to be comforted. I took another long deep breath and acknowledged that what I really needed was to feel. I nodded again, "I am ok," I thought.

SENSE

What are you feeling in your body right now? Put your hands on the sensation to locate where your feeling is being held.

I put both of my hands on my upper chest and neck and closed my eyes. My chest felt heavy. My throat felt thick and constricted. I inhaled through my nose, struggling to get a full breath past my throat and down into my dense lungs. Sad was trapped in me. Weighing down my chest, compressing my airway, and over flowing out my eyes. "Good," I could hear my coach in my mind. "Your chest feels heavy, your throat feels thick and constricted. You are ok. Breathe into that sensation." I exhaled and took another breath in.

EMOTION

What emotion are you feeling right now?

My mind drifted to *The 15 Commitments of Conscious Leadership*, which I had been reading. Commitment #3: Feel all Feelings.

I remembered that there were 5 primary emotions: anger, fear, sadness, joy, and sexual feelings. Today, at this moment, there was no doubt that sadness was calling to be felt. "Sad, I am feeling sad. It is ok to feel sad. I am ok," I whispered.

TAKE ACTION

The next step in feeling emotions is to allow them to physically move through the body.

I stood there, hands on my chest, tears flowing like a river, and repeated, "I feel sad. It is ok to feel sad. I am ok." My coach's voice floated back into my awareness, "Now, move. How does your sad want to move?" I walked over to the couch and curled up in the corner, wrapping my arms around my legs. Sad wanted to be rocked. I started rocking softly back and forth, allowing my body to bounce into the couch cushions.

HARMONIZE

Allow your feeling to be heard.

Tears flowed swiftly over my cheeks as a loud sob of grief escaped my throat. I squeezed my legs tighter and allowed my body to rock harder. Disappointment and despair wailed from my lungs as I rocked and cried. Wave after wave of sadness released from my body and escaped from my chest in convulsive gasps.

EXPRESS

Commit to releasing the emotion completely by expressing it through movement and sound until the sensation is fully resolved in your body.

I inhaled deeply; the air rushed in through my open throat, and the heaviness in my chest lifted with each howl. My arms relaxed and my body settled into a soft gentle rock. "Is there more?" I heard my coach's voice whisper in my mind. I let out a little whimper and sniffed my nose. I buried my face into my knees, my soft denim jeans soaking up the dwindling stream of tears. "I'm ok," I said as I exhaled, my whole body relaxing back onto the couch.

HUMAN

Congratulations! You are human!

"I'm ok. I'm ok. I'm ok." The reassuring mantra repeated over and over in my head. As I lay there on the couch, relaxed, my mind quiet, I realized that for the first time in a long time, I was ok. I inhaled slowly and let it out with a long sigh.

"I'm ok," I said out loud, nodding in agreement as I did.

UNPLUG

Unplug from the hustle of life.

As I sat there, hugged tenderly by the soft cushions of the couch, I reveled in those long, deep, nourishing breaths. It felt scary to lean into that ocean of sadness. Foreign to rock and wail and cry. But it was also the most free I had felt in a very long time. My chest was open; my breath deep and wide. My eyes roamed around the room and landed on the to-do lists laying innocently on the counter.

"What do you need right now?" I heard my coach's voice repeat in my mind.

Truth be told, I needed a timeout. A warm bath. A nap. A reboot.

SMILE

You just did the hardest thing of all. You chose to PAUSE THE HUSTLE and prioritize yourself.

I let out another soft breath and smiled.

I am okay.

For the first time in too long, I was okay. My smile stretched wider and brighter.

"Celebrate yourself!" I could hear my coach smiling as we celebrated this victory in my mind's eye.

I hadn't turned to chocolate or alcohol to numb. I hadn't soldiered on with my busyness. Instead, I had the courage to do the hardest thing of all: PAUSE, APPRECIATE myself in the moment, lean in, and UNDERSTAND that it was safe to feel. I located the SENSATION in my body, named the EMOTION, TOOK ACTION, and HARMONIZED with it until it was fully EXPRESSED. And now, here I was, a big SMILE on my face as I reflected on the progress I had made.

TRUST

You have always been and will always be your own best guide on this journey.

I thought back to the woman I was before coaching. The strong, dependable, badass that kept all the plates spinning and never allowed the positivity to crack. That badass persona was my protection and it was inflated in proportion to the pain I kept hidden behind the mask. I didn't trust myself. I thought that feelings were signs of weakness. All I knew was that my body was overweight and exhausted. All I knew was that my mind was overwhelmed and I was sick of the rat race. All I knew was that I was no longer willing to exist in this state of frenzied rushing; something had to change. I used to think that asking for help was only for the frail. Now, I know that asking for help just means I don't have to do the hard stuff alone. Through the tools that I currently provide for my clients, I learned how to trust myself again. I learned how to create safety within my experience so that I could begin feeling again. I learned how to put down the superhero cape and just be a human having a human experience.

LIBERATED

Learning to release feelings is your path to liberation.

The key to my self-imposed prison had been within me the whole time. Learning to feel my emotions through to completion set me free from binging, numbing, and distracting my way through life. Escaping the servitude to the superhero persona set me free to just be the one thing that I was always designed to be: uniquely, authentically, and unapologetically ME.

EMPOWERED

You have everything inside of yourself that you have ever needed.

If I could have done it on my own, I would have. If chocolate, alcohol, and being busy fixed it, I wouldn't have felt like such a mess. If the answer were somewhere outside of myself, I would never have any problems. But now that I know better, I can do better. Now that you know better, you can do better, too.

Breathe, my friend. You have faced fear, shame, guilt, and anger, and now you are already on the path to healing.

Real Talk

5-minute writing prompt:

Use the PAUSE THE HUSTLE practice to identify and process an emotion. Write about your experience.

Emotional release practice: We are emotional beings and learning to feel our feelings is a skill that can be practiced and mastered. Take a moment to PAUSE THE HUSTLE and practice.

Pro tip: We are ALWAYS FEELING SOMETHING.

- **P**AUSE: Pause, quiet the busy in your mind, and check in with yourself.
- **A**PPRECIATE: Appreciate this moment and know that it is OK to be where you are and to feel what you feel. Resist the urge to judge.
- **U**NDERSTAND: Understand that you are safe to feel your feelings
- **S**ENSE: What are you feeling in your body right now? Put your hands on the sensation to locate where your feeling is being held.
- **E**MOTION: What emotion are you feeling right now?
- **T**AKE ACTION: Go ahead; move, dance, contract, wiggle, kick, punch, rock, flail about.
- **H**ARMONIZE: Let it out! All those weird noises, let them out!
- **E**XPRESS: Commit to the process of expression until the feeling is fully released! When you think you are done, ask yourself, "Is there any more?"

Congratulate yourself for being **HUMAN**. You allowed yourself to **UNPLUG** from the seriousness of it all! **S**MILE! You did it! **T**RUST YOURSELF to be **LIBERATED** from suppressing your emotions and enjoy feeling **EMPOWERED** in your experience.

Reality Check

"Feelings are one of the universe's greatest gifts to human beings. They add richness and color to life. When emotions are understood (they are simply sensations occurring in and on the body), enjoyed and released (locate, describe, breathe, move, and vocalize), and wondered about with curiosity (what is this here to teach me?), they are a leader's essential ally." (Dethmer et al., 2014)[6]

Take Action

When I first started practicing the process of releasing my emotions, I found it difficult to even admit that I had an emotion, much less allow myself to feel. Having a coach in my corner was instrumental in supporting me to become friends with my feelings.

Full transparency, learning this skill is not something I can support you with in a free session. While you are always welcome to take advantage of the free coaching session, this work is accomplished over time, in baby steps, and is reserved for my one-on-one clients. Explore becoming a client and work directly with me. It's free to ask, and premium coaching is probably more affordable that you think!

---

[6] **Source:**
Dethmer, J. Chapman, D. Warner Klemp, K. The 15 Commitments of Conscious Leadership. 2014.

Scan QR code to schedule

https://linktr.cc/jessicasmithdossantos

MY WISH FOR YOU

Why did you become a Nurse?

I became a nurse because I love people.

Somewhere along the way I burned out. I fell out of love with serving. I stopped feeling good about what I did as a nurse. My soul felt dead and my life unfulfilled.

I became a nurse because I love people and I retired from nursing because I love people. Retirement was my way back to redeeming my love for those I serve and feeling fully alive and fulfilled in my life again.

My wish for you is that you feel loved, alive, aligned, and fulfilled so you can serve the world from a place of wholeness. You are not alone. Please know that you are free to live, love, and create a life around what matters most. May this life become alive, aligned, and fulfilled for you too.

————————————————————

My wish for you is that you feel loved,
alive, aligned, and fulfilled so you
can serve the world from a place of
wholeness. You are not alone. Please
know that you are free to live, love, and
create a life around what matters most.
May this life become alive, aligned, and
fulfilled for you too.

In the masterful words of the song "My Wish" by Rascal Flatts:

My wish, for you, is that this life becomes all that you want it to
Your dreams stay big, your worries stay small
You never need to carry more than you can hold
And while you're out there getting where you're getting to
I hope you know somebody loves you, and wants the same things too
Yeah, this, is my wish.

I see you. I hear you. I am you.

Through exams, books, and clinicals you did prepare
For every scenario this profession would dare
To test your resolve and push you to the brink
It will leave you wondering what to think.
"What did I get myself into? Was I remiss?
I thought this profession would be different than this."

I see you. I hear you. I am you.

Ooh nursing will test you, put you on your knees.
You will ask for a transfer just to appease
The anxiety in your chest, the doubt in your mind.
Yet, a few months later, you will wake up to find
Wherever you go, there you are.
Nothing can fix it, not even a stiff drink at the bar.
You will try to numb, to desensitize
You will wear the "happy nurse" mask, part of your disguise.
You will not be able to hide, because deep down inside,
Your soul will beg to be free, to be untied.

I see you. I hear you. I am you.

I know the burden in your heart and the weight in your shoes.
I know the ache in your chest as you deliver the news.
I see your hands, tired yet strong.
They work so hard to do no wrong.
The weight of the stethoscope that hangs from your neck.
You wonder how you became such a wreck.
The scars in your soul from the ones you have lost.
No one knows your pain or the terrible cost.

I see you. I hear you. I am you.

I know how you replay each scene in your mind.
Wondering what you missed, what you could have refined.
If you could do it again, would you do it differently?
It's too late now, you will never get to see.
Your eyes have cried endless tears
Thinking back on your career over the years.
Shifts so long you grew weary.
The times you felt dead inside, ghostly eerie.
The highs and the lows this profession will offer.
But the rest of the story, only you can author.
As the lows are counterbalanced by the highs
And your soul screams its angry cries.
No matter which department you will roam.
Inside yourself is your only true home.

I see you. I hear you. I am you.

Empowered with the skills to be your own caretaker
This profession will not be your deal breaker.
Armed with the pen of the past and the blank slate of the future
You will heal from the inside without needle or suture.
One second, one minute, one day at a time.
This life is not lost, you are still in your prime.
Let your heart hope for a better way.
I promise, my friend, there is still time in the day.
For you will learn to feel again.
Square your shoulders and raise up your chin.
You are a nurse; you do hard things.
You are not broken and you do not need strings
To tie yourself together, to push through the pain
You have nothing more to lose and everything to gain.
There is nowhere to go but up from here.
So, dry your eyes, take my hand, do not fear.
You got this, you can, now surrender your soul.
You are and have always been, the one in control.

I see you. I hear you. I am you.

HOW CAN I SERVE YOU?

In the loving words of my coach, "If you could do it alone, you would have done it already." Those words may have stepped on my toes and bruised my pride, but I could not argue with the truth in her statement.

Saying yes to partnering with a coach and leaning into a community of others wanting better for their lives was exactly what I needed to move forward with my healing. Now, it is my responsibility to pay it forward. I know there are far too many Nurses in this world that are suffering from the burdens of shame, guilt, fear, sadness, and anger in the same ways I was. My mission is to empower nurses to feel loved, alive, aligned, and fulfilled so they can serve the world from a place of wholeness.

Now I ask you, are you ready to lock elbows with a partner in your health and healing?

Let's Connect

- Join us in the Sh*t They Don't Tell You In Nursing School community. We would all love the opportunity to get to know you more.
- Follow me on social media for tips, stories, inspiration, and recipes.
- Schedule a free coaching call with me.

Let's Team Up

- **Become a client:** My clients receive an individualized holistic coaching program. Together, we will explore all the options and find a financially friendly plan that is customized to your physical and mental health goals.
- **Become a referral partner:** You know nurses that I don't know. I pay you for connecting me to the nurses in your world that may need to feel loved, alive, aligned, and fulfilled again.
- **Become a coaching partner:** The mission to see nurses serving from a place of wholeness is not just a "me" job, it is a "we" job! I am always looking to mentor new coach partners who would love to generate an income stream by supporting nurses to create alive, aligned, and fulfilled lives.

If I can turn my hurt into healing, and feel alive, fulfilled, and fully aligned again, there is hope for you too. Until the next perfect time!

Much Love,

Coach Jess

Scan QR code to for more

https://linktr.ee/jessicasmithdossantos

Made in the USA
Las Vegas, NV
27 January 2024